DEPRESSO

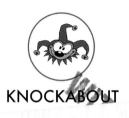

KNOCKABOUT

DEPRESSO

or: How I Learned To Stop Worrying...

And Embrace Being Bonkers!

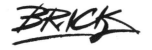

Depresso

© 2010 by John Stuart Clark

Published by Knockabout Limited
119 Roundwood Road
London NW10 9UL
United Kingdom
www.knockabout.com

Design and Layout by Romain Janicki

John Stuart Clark (Brick) has asserted his right
under the Copyright, Designs and Patents Act
1988 to be identified as the author of this work..
All rights reserved.

No part of this book may be reproduced, stored in
the retrieval system or transmitted in any form
without the prior permission of the publisher or
copyright holder.

A CIP catalogue record for this book is available
from the British Library.

ISBN 9780861661701

Printed in China

First Printing

CONTENTS

 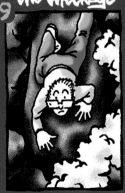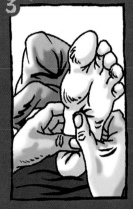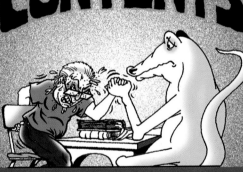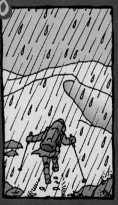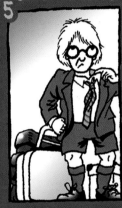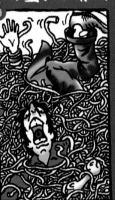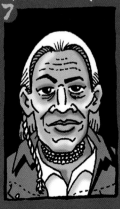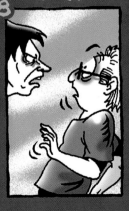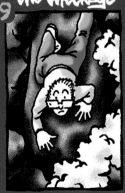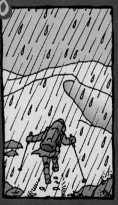

EXCEPT THAT I SMOKED A HANDFUL OF ROLL-UPS A DAY, I WAS LUDICROUSLY **FIT** FOR MY AGE.

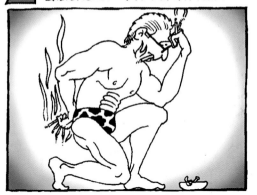

I SWAM AND WALKED AND CLIMBED, EVEN POTHOLED OCCASIONALLY, AND I CYCLED **EVERYWHERE**. A 30 MILE ROUND TRIP TO DROP IN ON PALS DIDN'T FAZE ME.

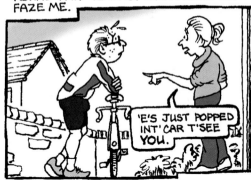

'E'S JUST POPPED INT' CAR T'SEE YOU.

(HELL, A COUPLE OF YEARS EARLIER I HAD PEDALLED ACROSS AMERICA, EAST TO WEST, **INTO** THE GODDAMN WIND.)

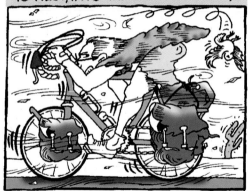

I ATE HEALTHILY, SLEPT OKAY, SOCIALISED WELL AND WORKED HARD AT A JOB I LOVED.

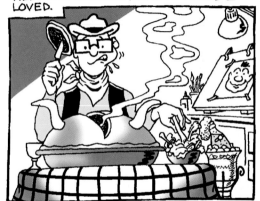

AND I LOVED WELL. IN FACT I WAS SEXUALLY **IRREPRESSIBLE**, WITH AN UNREASONABLE RECOVERY RATE.

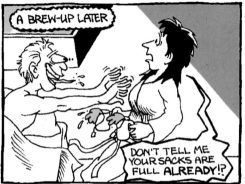

A BREW-UP LATER

DON'T TELL ME YOUR SACKS ARE FULL ALREADY!?

I HADN'T SUFFERED SO MUCH AS A COLD IN TWENTY YEARS, SO WHEN IT HIT, IT HIT **HARD**.

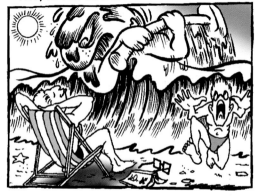

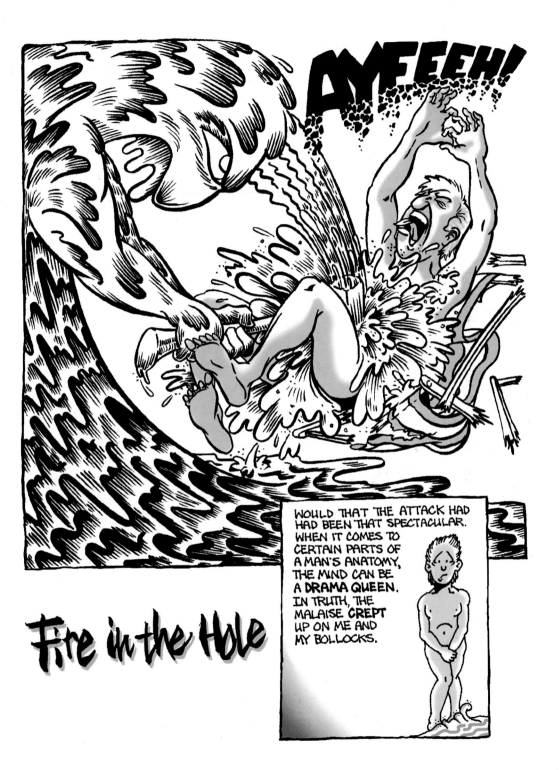

AYEEEH!

Fire in the Hole

WOULD THAT THE ATTACK HAD HAD BEEN THAT SPECTACULAR. WHEN IT COMES TO CERTAIN PARTS OF A MAN'S ANATOMY, THE MIND CAN BE A **DRAMA QUEEN.** IN TRUTH, THE MALAISE **CREPT** UP ON ME AND MY BOLLOCKS.

AT FIRST IT WAS A DULL ACHE AND MILD SUSPICION THAT FOUND ME ROOTING THROUGH OFFICE PAPERS.

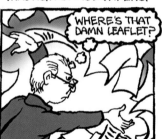

WHERE'S THAT DAMN LEAFLET?

FOLLOWING MY HEALTH CENTRE'S STEP-BY-STEP GUIDE, I CHECKED FOR TELL-TALE SIGNS.

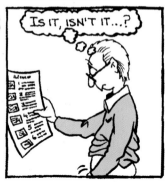

IS IT, ISN'T IT...?

I WAS **CLEAR**, BUT WITHIN A COUPLE OF WEEKS THE DULL ACHE HAD BECOME A DEEPLY SUSPICIOUS **THROB**. MY INVESTIGATION TECHNIQUES WENT HI-TECH. I EMPLOYED A MIRROR.

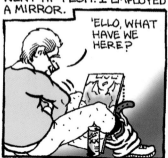

'ELLO, WHAT HAVE WE HERE?

ONE BOLLOCK WAS SIGNIFICANTLY LARGER THAN THE OTHER; AS DIFFERENT AS A SQUISHY PEA TO A SOLID CUE BALL.

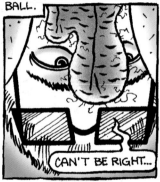

CAN'T BE RIGHT...

BANG BANG

WHAT ARE YOU DOING IN THERE, TOM? I NEED A WAZ...

JUST ER... CLIPPING MY TOE NAILS.

I HAD KEPT MY FEARS FROM MY PARTNER BECAUSE, WELL, REAL MEN DO. WHAT WOULD I SAY?

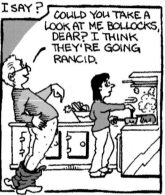

COULD YOU TAKE A LOOK AT ME BOLLOCKS, DEAR? I THINK THEY'RE GOING RANCID.

BUT JUDY BECAME SUSPICIOUS.

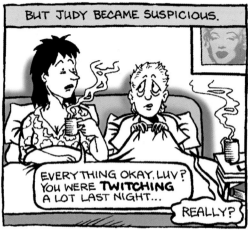

EVERYTHING OKAY, LUV? YOU WERE **TWITCHING** A LOT LAST NIGHT...

REALLY?

TOO RIGHT I WAS!! ELECTRIC EELS WERE PLAYING VOLLEYBALL WITH MY GONADS IN A SUB-ARCTIC SEA, OR SO IT FELT.

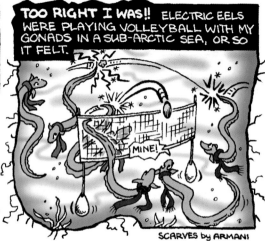

MINE!

SCARVES BY ARMANI

ON THE PRETEXT THAT JUDY WAS SNORING LIKE A MARE *, I MOVED INTO THE SPARE ROOM TO SUFFER WITHOUT FUSS.

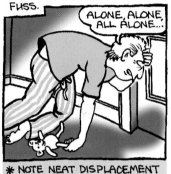

ALONE, ALONE, ALL ALONE...

* NOTE NEAT DISPLACEMENT OF BLAME.

LIKE ICE ON FLESH, THE SENSATION IN MY CRUTCH QUIETLY MUTATED FROM FREEZING COLD TO BURNING HOT. I COULD HAVE GRILLED MARSHMALLOWS.

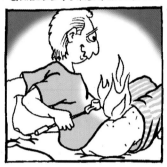

THE SHOOTING PAINS INTENSIFIED BUT I FORCED MYSELF TO FOCUS ON OTHER MATTERS.

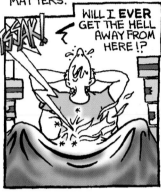

WILL I EVER GET THE HELL AWAY FROM HERE!?

TSSAK!

WE WERE SELLING UP AND MOVING HOUSE, EXCEPT WE HADN'T SOLD OR AGREED WHERE TO MOVE TO.

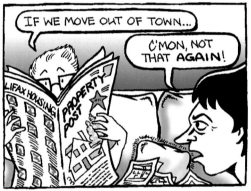

IF WE MOVE OUT OF TOWN...

C'MON, NOT THAT AGAIN!

HALIFAX HOUSING

PROPERTY POST

LOOK, WE STAY AROUND HERE WE'RE LOCKED INTO THE SAME OLD MEDIOCRE SCENE.

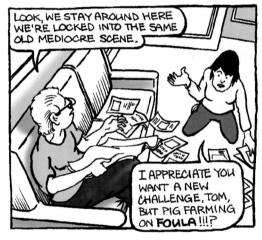

I APPRECIATE YOU WANT A NEW CHALLENGE, TOM, BUT PIG FARMING ON FOULA!!!?

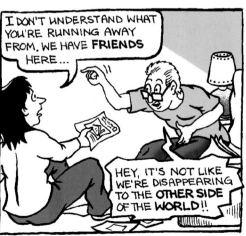

I DON'T UNDERSTAND WHAT YOU'RE RUNNING AWAY FROM. WE HAVE FRIENDS HERE...

HEY, IT'S NOT LIKE WE'RE DISAPPEARING TO THE OTHER SIDE OF THE WORLD!!

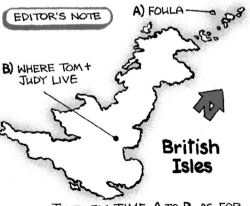

EDITOR'S NOTE

A) FOULA

B) WHERE TOM + JUDY LIVE

British Isles

JOURNEY TIME A TO B, AS FOR FLIGHT FROM TOKYO TO LONDON.

9

I ADMIT IT, I WAS **DESPERATE** TO MOVE AWAY.

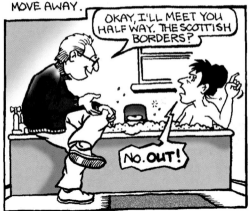

OKAY, I'LL MEET YOU HALF WAY. THE SCOTTISH BORDERS?

NO. OUT!

I WAS PACKED **EIGHT MONTHS** BEFORE THE 'FOR SALE' SIGN WENT UP.

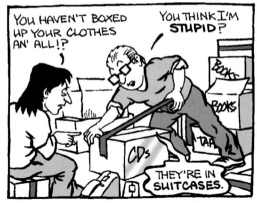

YOU HAVEN'T BOXED UP YOUR CLOTHES AN' ALL!?

YOU THINK I'M **STUPID?**

THEY'RE IN SUITCASES.

AUGUST

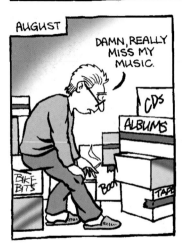

DAMN, REALLY MISS MY MUSIC.

NOVEMBER

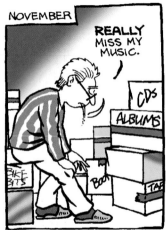

REALLY MISS MY MUSIC.

FEBRUARY

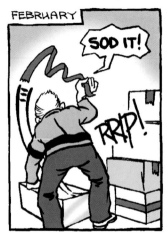

SOD IT!

RRIP!

FOR MONTHS I LIVED IN A **MESS** OF RIFLED BOXES.

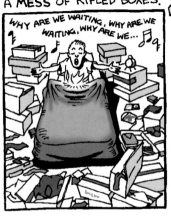

WHY ARE WE WAITING, WHY ARE WE WAITING, WHY ARE WE...

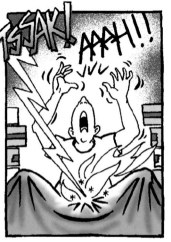

TSSAK!

AAAH!!!

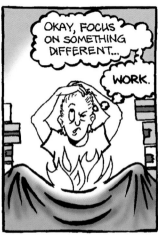

OKAY, FOCUS ON SOMETHING DIFFERENT...

WORK.

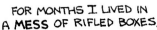

ACCEPTING THAT I WAS NEVER GOING TO BE THE NEXT KEITH RICHARDS, THE JOB I STUMBLED INTO WAS A **COOL** CONSOLATION PRIZE. WHEN PEOPLE ASKED I TOLD THEM...

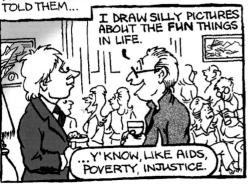

I DRAW SILLY PICTURES ABOUT THE **FUN** THINGS IN LIFE.

...Y'KNOW, LIKE AIDS, POVERTY, INJUSTICE.

SURPRISINGLY, IT **WASN'T** A CONVERSATION STOPPER.

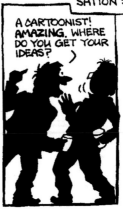

A CARTOONIST! **AMAZING.** WHERE DO YOU GET YOUR IDEAS?

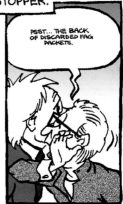

PSST... THE BACK OF DISCARDED FAG PACKETS.

IN A WORLD RUN BY **LUNATIC PEOPLE** FOR **LUNATIC PURPOSES**, I LIKED TO THINK I WAS STRIKING A BLOW FOR **SANITY**, IF ONLY MY OWN.

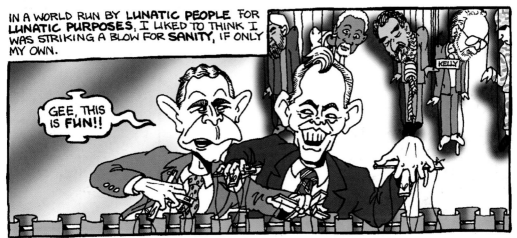

GEE, THIS IS **FUN**!!

KELLY

FROM AN EARLY AGE I STOOD ASIDE FROM THE CROWD AND MUTTERED, 'BAH, HUMBUG!', SOMETIMES A LITTLE TOO LOUD.

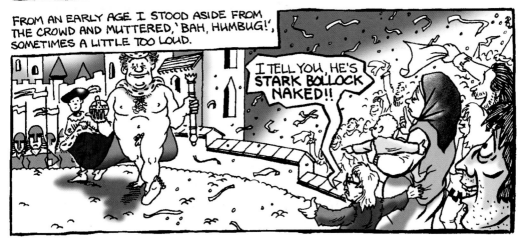

I TELL YOU HE'S STARK BOLLOCK NAKED!!

11

BUT OF LATE THE LUNACY HAD WORN GROUND ME DOWN. THE **BULLSHIT** WAS NO LONGER FUNNY...

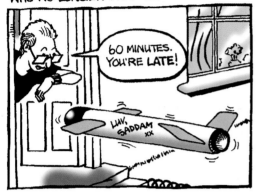

THE **HYPOCRICY** NO LONGER RISIBLE...

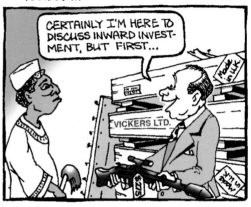

AND THE **INIQUITIES** HAD GONE FAR BEYOND FARCICAL.

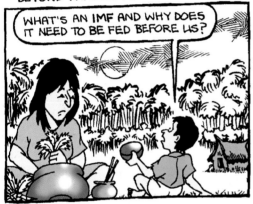

BUT WHAT REALLY BUGGED ME WAS THAT NOBODY **GAVE A TOSS** ANYMORE.

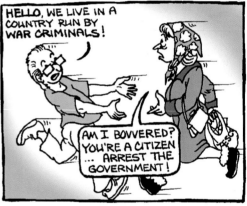

... OR IF THEY DID, THEY DISGUISED THEIR OUTRAGE WITH **CYNICISM**.

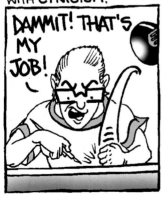

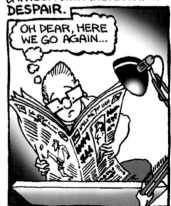

I APPROACHED EACH NEW CARTOON WITH INCREASING **DESPAIR**.

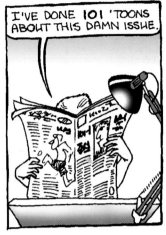

I'VE DONE **101** 'TOONS ABOUT THIS DAMN ISSUE.

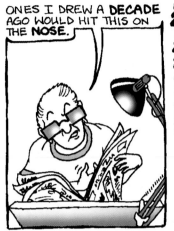

ONES I DREW A **DECADE** AGO WOULD HIT THIS ON THE **NOSE.**

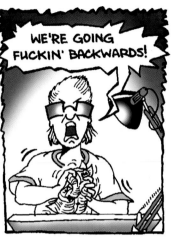

WE'RE GOING FUCKIN' BACKWARDS!

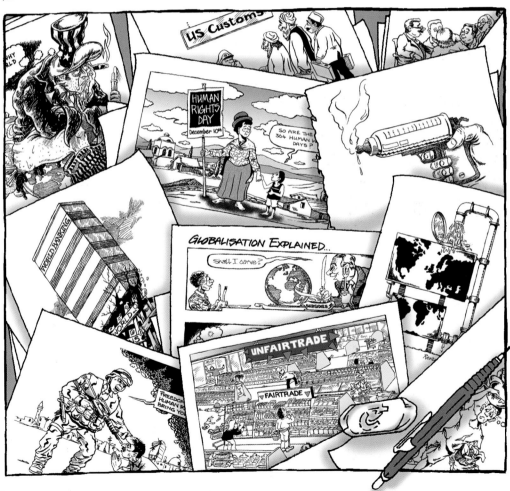

13

THEN THE **KILLER BLOW** WAS STRUCK.

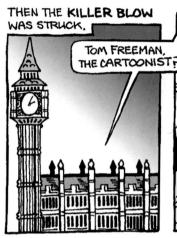

TOM FREEMAN, THE CARTOONIST?

HI, I'M P.A. TO THE RIGHT HONORABLE...

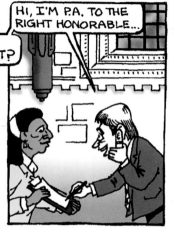

WHAT, LIKE BERNARD TO JIM HACKER?

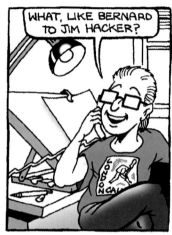

NO, I DON'T SUPPOSE THAT IS FUNNY...

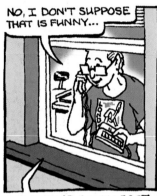

HE DOES!? SO AT LEAST YOUR MINISTER HAS A SENSE OF HUMOUR.

YES, WELL HE WOULD LIKE TO PURCHASE THE ORIGINAL OF...

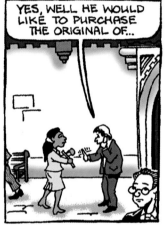

BUT I DEPICTED HIM AS A...

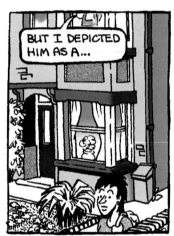

...A LOYAL KNIGHT?

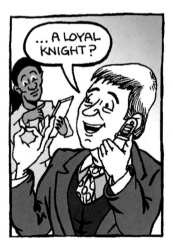

I'D HAVE SAID 'TOADY'...

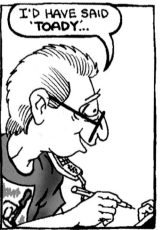

WHATEVER. IS IT FOR SALE AND WHAT'S YOUR PRICE?

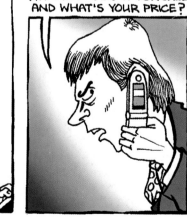

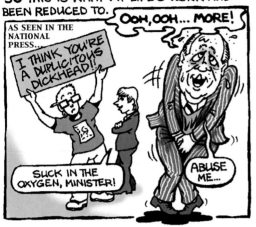

SO THIS IS WHAT MY LIFE'S WORK HAD BEEN REDUCED TO.

AS SEEN IN THE NATIONAL PRESS...

I THINK YOU'RE A DUPLICITOUS DICKHEAD!

SUCK IN THE OXYGEN, MINISTER!

OOH, OOH... MORE!

ABUSE ME...

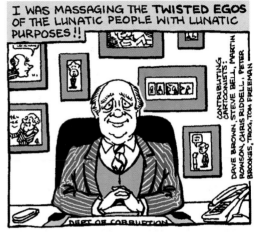

I WAS MASSAGING THE **TWISTED EGOS** OF THE LUNATIC PEOPLE WITH LUNATIC PURPOSES!!

CONTRIBUTING CARTOONISTS: DAVE BROWN, STEVE BELL, MARTIN ROWSON, CHRIS RIDDELL, PETER BROOKES, TROG, TOM FREEMAN

DEPT OF CORRUPTION

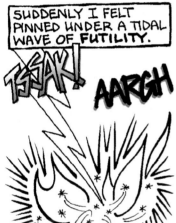

SUDDENLY I FELT PINNED UNDER A TIDAL WAVE OF **FUTILITY**.

TSSAK!

AARGH

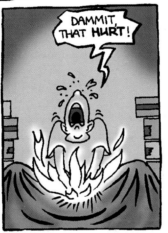

DAMMIT, THAT **HURT**!

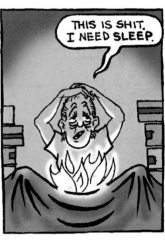

THIS IS SHIT. I NEED SLEEP.

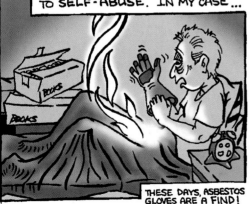

AT THIS POINT THE MALE OF THE SPECIES GENERALLY RESORTS TO SELF-ABUSE. IN MY CASE...

BOOKS

BOOKS

THESE DAYS, ASBESTOS GLOVES ARE A FIND!

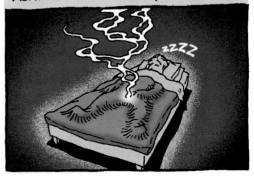

THIS WENT ON FOR SEVERAL MONTHS, NOT A NIGHT OF IT SPENT WITH JUDY. THE LAST TIME I EXPERIENCED SUCH MONUMENTAL CELIBACY, I HAD ACNE.

ZZZZ

15

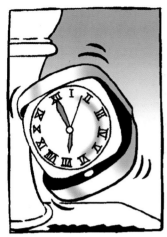
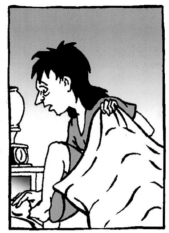
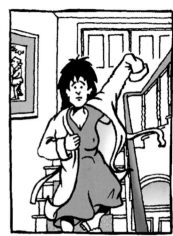
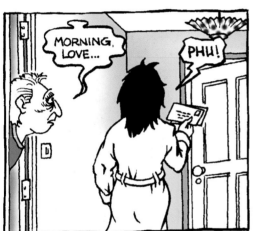
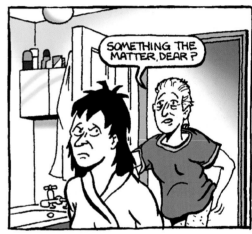
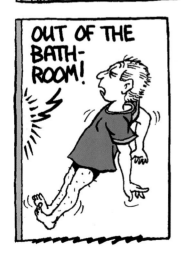
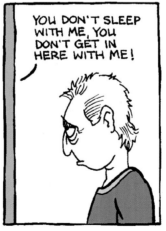
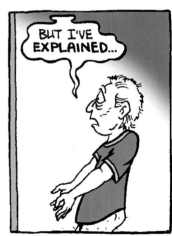

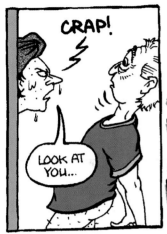

CRAP!

LOOK AT YOU...

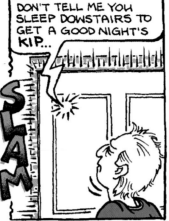

DON'T TELL ME YOU SLEEP DOWSTAIRS TO GET A GOOD NIGHT'S KIP...

SLAM

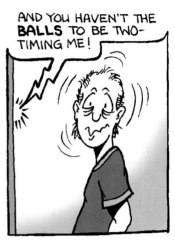

AND YOU HAVEN'T THE **BALLS** TO BE TWO-TIMING ME!

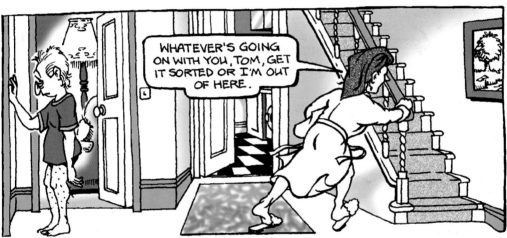

WHATEVER'S GOING ON WITH YOU, TOM, GET IT SORTED OR I'M OUT OF HERE.

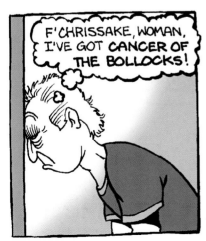

F'CHRISSAKE, WOMAN, I'VE GOT **CANCER OF THE BOLLOCKS!**

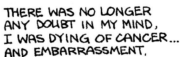

THERE WAS NO LONGER ANY DOUBT IN MY MIND, I WAS DYING OF CANCER... AND EMBARRASSMENT.

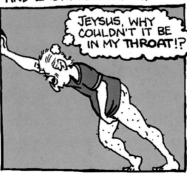

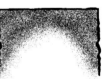

JEYSUS, WHY COULDN'T IT BE IN MY **THROAT**!?

I DECIDED TO FACE UP TO THE BAD NEWS AND GO TO THE DOCTOR...

NEXT WEEK.

17

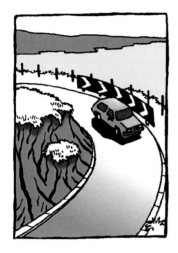

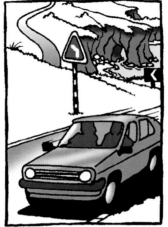

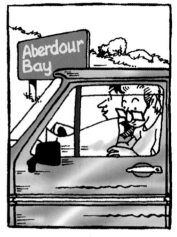

STRANGELY ENOUGH, I NEVER HAD A PROBLEM WITH MY BOLLOCKS DURING THE DAY – NO PANGS, TWANGS OR BURNING.

MY URINE REEKED OF CORIANDER AND MY CRAPS WERE INDUSTRIAL STRENGTH, BUT OTHERWISE I FELT FAIRLY NORMAL.

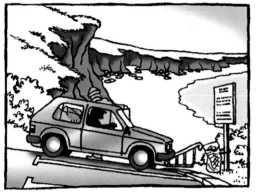

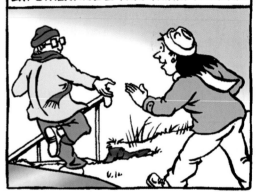

YES, I WANTED TO FLEE MY HOME TOWN AND FOUND WORK REPUGNANT, BUT OTHERWISE...

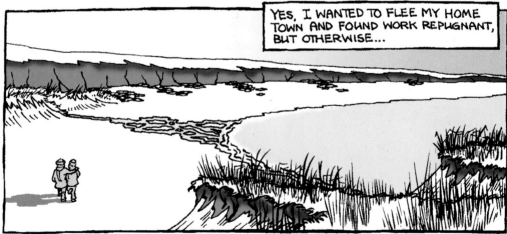

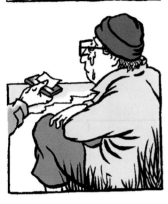

OKAY... THERE **WERE** OTHER PROBLEMS...

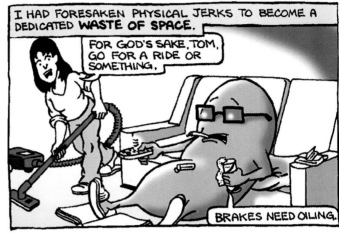

I HAD FORESAKEN PHYSICAL JERKS TO BECOME A DEDICATED **WASTE OF SPACE.**

FOR GOD'S SAKE, TOM, GO FOR A RIDE OR SOMETHING.

BRAKES NEED OILING.

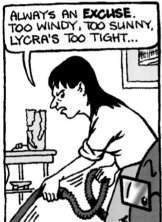

ALWAYS AN **EXCUSE.** TOO WINDY, TOO SUNNY, LYCRA'S TOO TIGHT...

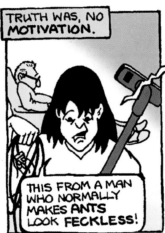

TRUTH WAS, NO **MOTIVATION.**

THIS FROM A MAN WHO NORMALLY MAKES ANTS LOOK FECKLESS!

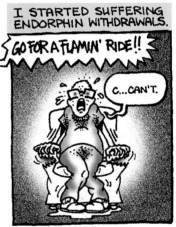

I STARTED SUFFERING ENDORPHIN WITHDRAWALS.

GO FOR A FLAMIN' RIDE!!

C...CAN'T.

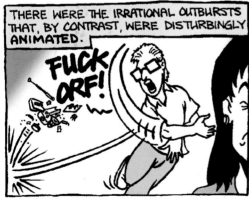

THERE WERE THE IRRATIONAL OUTBURSTS THAT, BY CONTRAST, WERE DISTURBINGLY ANIMATED.

FUCK ORF!

WE GOT THROUGH A LOT OF RADIOS, PARTICULARLY DURING THE 'TODAY' PROGRAMME.

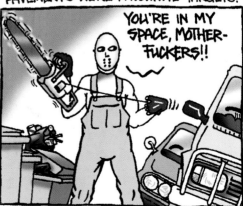

CARS AND WHEELIE BINS PARKED ON PAVEMENTS WERE FAVOURITE TARGETS.

YOU'RE IN MY SPACE, MOTHER-FUCKERS!!

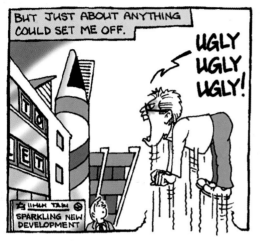

BUT JUST ABOUT ANYTHING COULD SET ME OFF.

UGLY UGLY UGLY!

SPARKLING NEW DEVELOPMENT

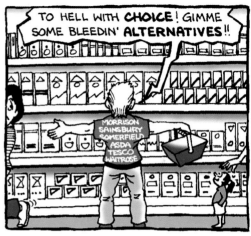

TO HELL WITH **CHOICE**! GIMME SOME BLEEDIN' **ALTERNATIVES**!!

MORRISON SAINSBURY SOMERFIELD ASDA TESCO WAITROSE

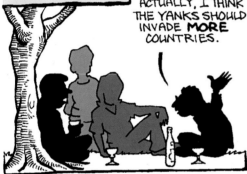

THEN THERE WAS MY **HUMOUR**. ACERBIC AT THE BEST OF TIMES, FRIENDS WERE USED TO MY UNCOMFORTABLE WIT. IT WENT WITH THE JOB.

ACTUALLY, I THINK THE YANKS SHOULD INVADE **MORE** COUNTRIES.

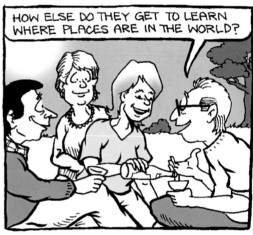

HOW ELSE DO THEY GET TO LEARN WHERE PLACES ARE IN THE WORLD?

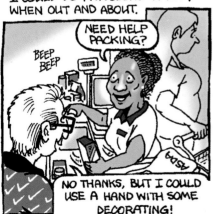

I COULD DO FRIVOLOUS 'N ALL, WHEN OUT AND ABOUT.

NEED HELP PACKING?

BEEP BEEP

NO THANKS, BUT I COULD USE A HAND WITH SOME DECORATING!

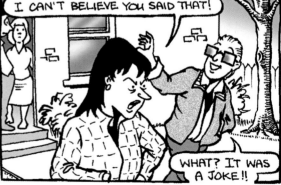

BUT LATELY MY HUMOUR HAD BECOME BITTER AND TWISTED. I NO LONGER POKED FUN. I **NUKED**.

I CAN'T BELIEVE YOU SAID THAT!

WHAT? IT WAS A JOKE!!

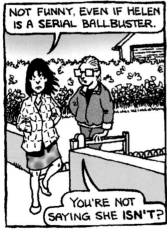

NOT FUNNY, EVEN IF HELEN IS A **SERIAL BALLBUSTER**.

YOU'RE NOT SAYING SHE **ISN'T**?

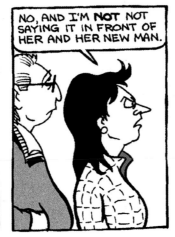

NO, AND I'M **NOT** NOT SAYING IT IN FRONT OF HER AND HER NEW MAN.

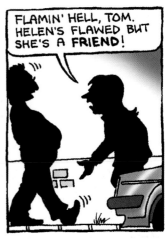

FLAMIN' HELL, TOM. HELEN'S FLAWED BUT SHE'S A **FRIEND**!

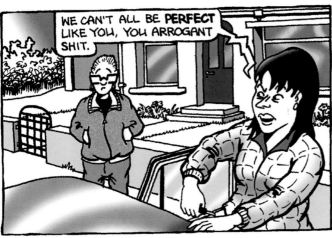

WE CAN'T ALL BE **PERFECT** LIKE YOU, YOU ARROGANT SHIT.

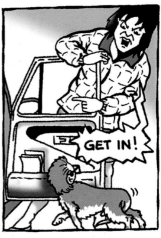

GET IN!

THAT WAS THE **PITS**. FOR SOME BIZARRE REASON, I WAS HELL BENT ON ALIENATING OUR FRIENDS.

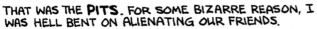

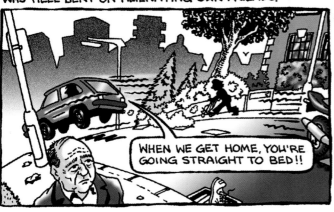

WHEN WE GET HOME, YOU'RE GOING STRAIGHT TO BED!!

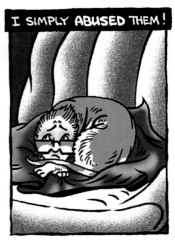

I SIMPLY **ABUSED** THEM!

21

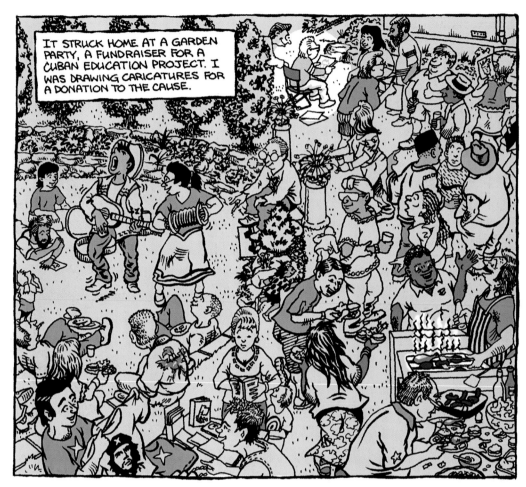

IT STRUCK HOME AT A GARDEN PARTY, A FUNDRAISER FOR A CUBAN EDUCATION PROJECT. I WAS DRAWING CARICATURES FOR A DONATION TO THE CAUSE.

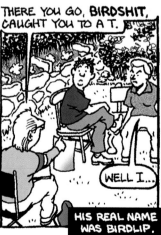

THERE YOU GO, **BIRDSHIT**, CAUGHT YOU TO A T.

WELL I...

HIS REAL NAME WAS BIRDLIP.

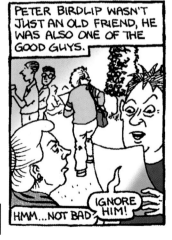

PETER BIRDLIP WASN'T JUST AN OLD FRIEND, HE WAS ALSO ONE OF THE GOOD GUYS.

HMM...NOT BAD

IGNORE HIM!

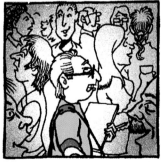

AT A GATHERING STIFF WITH CREEPY LIBERALS AND WEEK-END RADICALS, PETER WAS THE REAL THING AND THE **LEAST** DESERVING OF MY...

MY **ANGER**, I SUPPOSE.

I TOOK FLIGHT. I WANTED TO **BEAT THE CRAP** OUT OF ME, DIG A SHALLOW GRAVE.

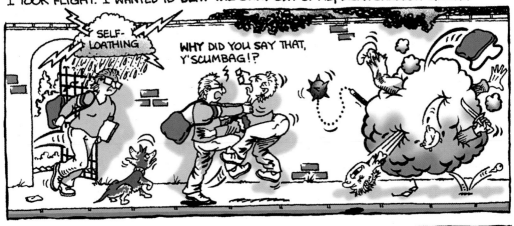

INSTEAD, I CONVINCED MYSELF I HAD NO FRIENDS.

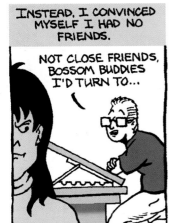

NOT CLOSE FRIENDS, BOSSOM BUDDIES I'D TURN TO...

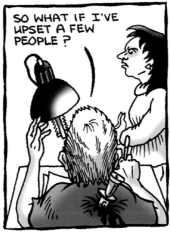

SO WHAT IF I'VE UPSET A FEW PEOPLE?

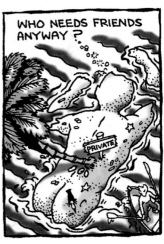

WHO NEEDS FRIENDS ANYWAY?

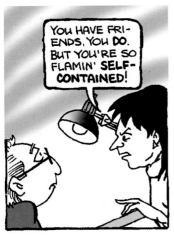

YOU HAVE FRIENDS, YOU **DO**. BUT YOU'RE SO FLAMIN' **SELF-CONTAINED!**

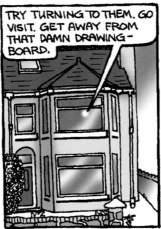

TRY TURNING TO THEM. GO VISIT. GET AWAY FROM THAT DAMN DRAWING-BOARD.

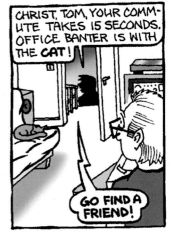

CHRIST, TOM, YOUR COMMUTE TAKES 15 SECONDS. OFFICE BANTER IS WITH THE **CAT**!

GO FIND A FRIEND!

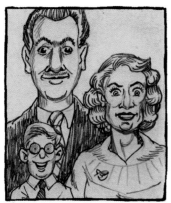

I WAS A SINGLE KID BORN OF SINGLE KIDS.

OUR FAMILY TREE RAN STRAIGHT UP AND DOWN.

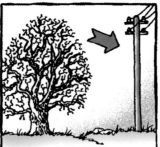

I STILL COULDN'T TELL YOU WHAT A NEPHEW OR COUSIN IS WITHOUT CHECKING A DICTIONARY.

ANY CHANCE OF THE FREEMANS GRAFTING ON BRANCHES FROM A FAMILY OF FIRM FRIENDS WAS FRUSTRATED BY MOVING EVERY THREE YEARS, GENERALLY TO ANOTHER **COUNTRY**.

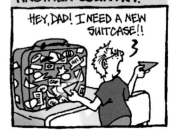

HEY, DAD! I NEED A NEW SUITCASE!!

I SPENT A LOT OF TIME ON MY OWNSOME...

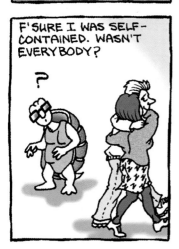

WHICH MEANT A LOT OF TIME IN MY HEAD, MAYBE MORE THAN WAS **HEALTHY**.

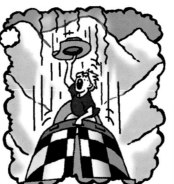

CROSSING DESERTS ON MY OWN WAS A NATURAL PROGRESSION.

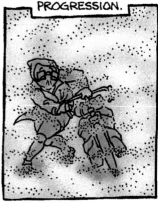

F'SURE I WAS SELF-CONTAINED. WASN'T EVERYBODY?

?

WHAT HAD FRIENDS AND FAMILY TO DO WITH ANYTHING?

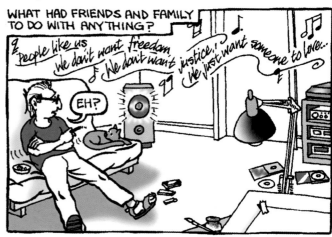

People like us we don't want freedom. We don't want justice, we just want someone to love...

EH?

24

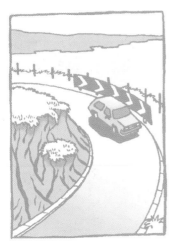

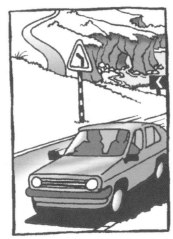

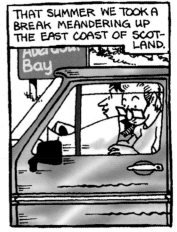

That summer we took a break meandering up the east coast of Scotland.

It was the first trip we'd ever done that didn't have an agenda, an itinerary.

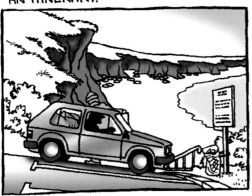

We just drifted for a fortnight.

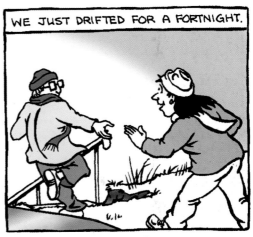

What Scotland lacks in tropical sunshine it makes up in sublime head space.

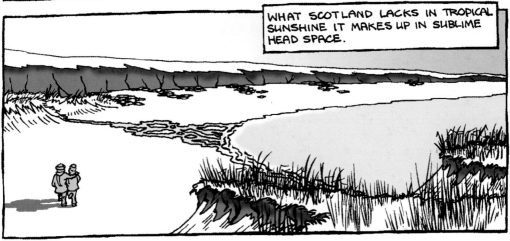

AS THE MORPHIN STRUGGLES TO CONTAIN THE AGONY OF THE CANCER'S FINAL ONSLAUGHT...

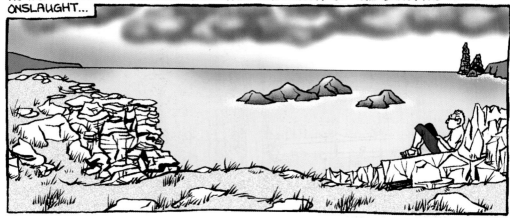

PRAY GOD I FIND A QUIET CORNER AMIDST THE PANIC WHERE I CAN TARRY.

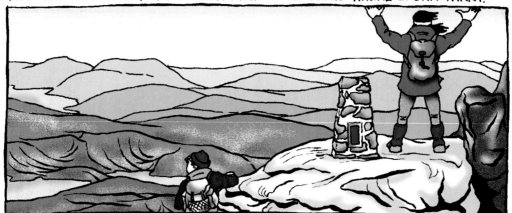

BY THEN I MIGHT HAVE GOT RELIGION, BUT JUST IN CASE, I WAS STORING UP REMEMBERANCES.

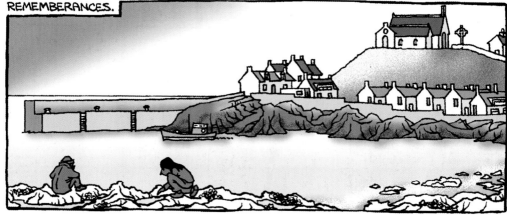

BUT SOME PLACES WERE DEPRESSING. LIKE FRASERBURGH. YOU COULD **SMELL** THE RAVAGES OF THE BRUSSELS PLAGUE.

DEATH WAFTED ROUND THE COLD STONE STREETS OF EVERY HARBOUR TOWN — DEATH AND BEWILDERMENT.

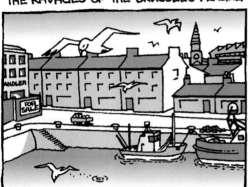

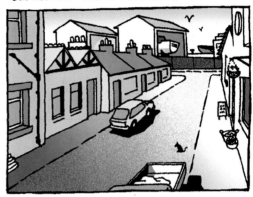

AS ONE OLD SALT TOLD US...

WE COULD BE THE ONLY ISLAND IN THE WORLD WITHOUT A FISHING INDUSTRY.

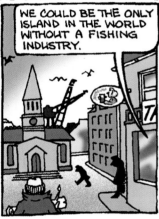

ANOTHER SUCCESSFUL PACIFICATION BY WESTMINSTER.

WHO NEVER GOT OVER BANNOCK-BURN...

WHO LET BRUSSELS PISS ALL OVER US!!

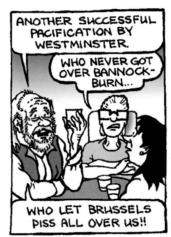

BUT Y' KNOW, WE'VE STILL GOT THE **WHISKY!**

SO ALL'S NOT LOST?

MY ROUND.

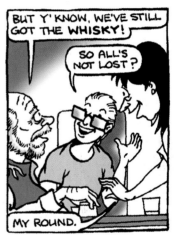

IT'S TRUE. ALL THE GOLD IN THE BANK OF ENGLAND COULDN'T BUY THE SCOTTISH SCOTCH RESERVES.

REALLY?

WHY DO YOU THINK THEY TAX IT TO HELL AND BACK!?

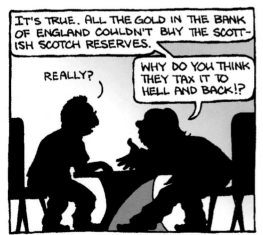

SLUAGH GHAIRM!

The Thistle

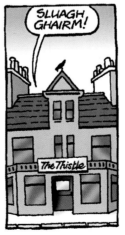

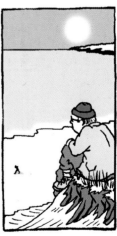

27

I DID A LOT OF COGITATING THAT SUMMER. I COGITATED IN FRONT OF FIRES...

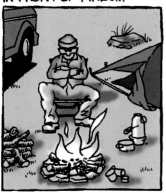

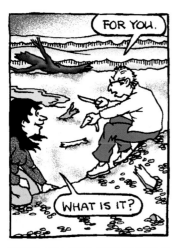

FISHING NETS...

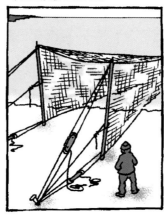

AND A BIT OF DRIFTWOOD, WITH A KNIFE.

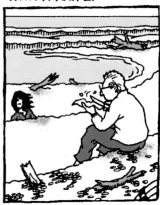

FOR YOU.

WHAT IS IT?

DUNNO. THIS SIDE IT'S A DOLPHIN. THAT IT'S A LIZARD.

IS THAT WHAT YOU'VE BEEN WHITTLING ALL ALL THIS TIME?

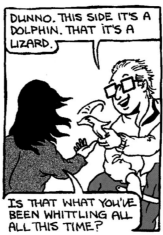

I'VE BEEN THINKING.

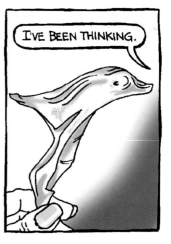

I OWE A LOT OF PEOPLE AN APOLOGY.

YOU DO.

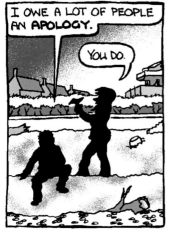

I'VE BEEN A DICKHEAD, PARTICULARLY WITH YOU.

YEP.

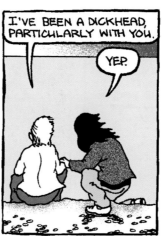

AND...?

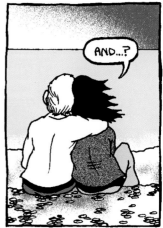

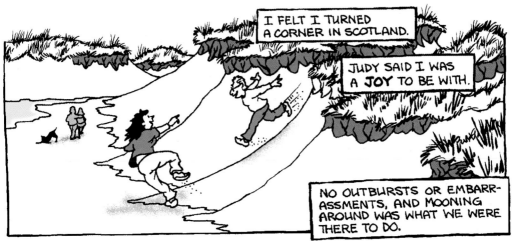

I FELT I TURNED A CORNER IN SCOTLAND.

JUDY SAID I WAS A **JOY** TO BE WITH.

NO OUTBURSTS OR EMBARR-ASSMENTS, AND MOONING AROUND WAS WHAT WE WERE THERE TO DO.

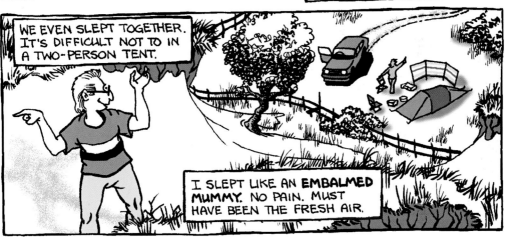

WE EVEN SLEPT TOGETHER. IT'S DIFFICULT NOT TO IN A TWO-PERSON TENT.

I SLEPT LIKE AN **EMBALMED MUMMY**. NO PAIN. MUST HAVE BEEN THE FRESH AIR.

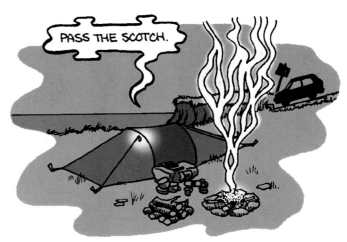

PASS THE SCOTCH.

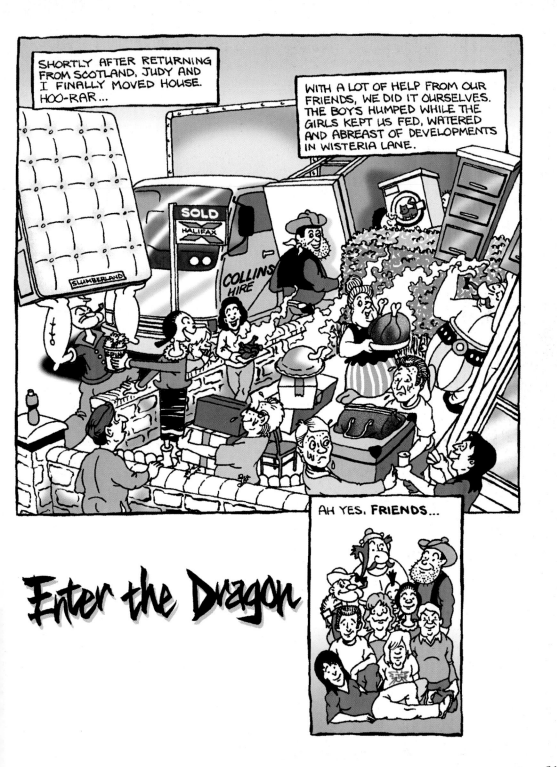

Enter the Dragon

WE MOVED
FROM THIS...

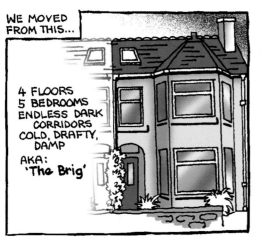

4 FLOORS
5 BEDROOMS
ENDLESS DARK
  CORRIDORS
COLD, DRAFTY,
  DAMP

AKA:
'The Brig'

TO THIS...

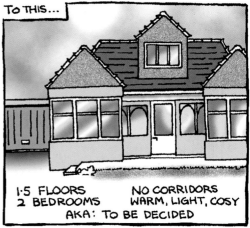

1.5 FLOORS   NO CORRIDORS
2 BEDROOMS   WARM, LIGHT, COSY
         AKA: TO BE DECIDED

WE HAD REACHED A COMPROMISE ON WHICH
PART OF THE COUNTRY TO MOVE TO.

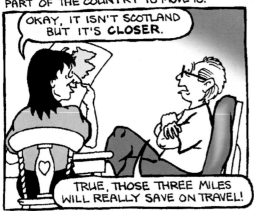

OKAY, IT ISN'T SCOTLAND
BUT IT'S **CLOSER.**

TRUE, THOSE THREE MILES
WILL REALLY SAVE ON TRAVEL!

WE RELOCATED
FROM THE LITTER
STREWN INNER
CITY...

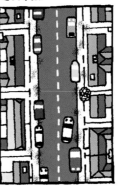

TO LEAF STREWN
SUBURBIA...

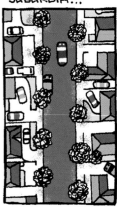

... WHERE IT SEEMED RESIDENTS VARNISHED THEIR
CARS AND IRONED LAWNS AT LEAST ONCE A WEEK.

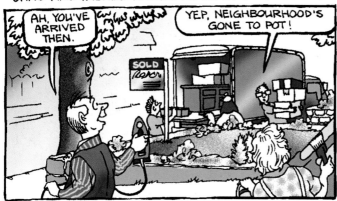

AH, YOU'VE
ARRIVED
THEN.

YEP, NEIGHBOURHOOD'S
GONE TO POT!

SOLD

I COULDN'T PUT THE OLD
PLACE BEHIND ME FAST
ENOUGH, BUT WAS LESS
THAN CONVINCED BY
THE NEW.

WHY DO I
FEEL LIKE A MILK-
MAN RETIRED TO
SKEGNESS!?

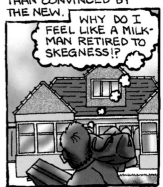

ITS ONE REDEEMING FEATURE WAS A BACKLINE OF LEYLANDII THAT BLOCKED OUT THE WORLD.

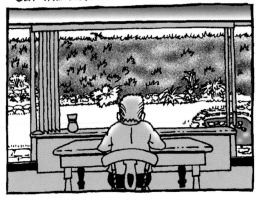

OH, AND A POND WITH AN INDETERMINATE NUMBER OF HYPERACTIVE GOLDFISH THAT KEPT ME OCCUPIED FOR DAYS.

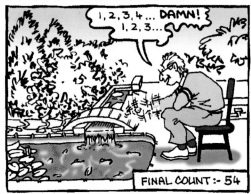

1, 2, 3, 4... DAMN! 1, 2, 3...

FINAL COUNT :- 54

I MADE A BIG EFFORT. BEFORE WE WERE EVEN UNPACKED, I SAT DOWN TO WRITE APOLOGIES TO EVERYBODY I'D PISSED OFF IN RECENT MONTHS.

THE LIST WAS LONG.

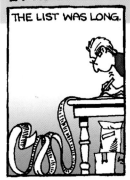

I WHITTLED IT DOWN...

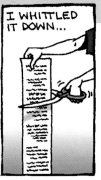

AND MANAGED THREE LETTERS BEFORE THE REPETITION OF MY SINS BECAME **DEPRESSING**.

JESUS, WORRA TOSSER!

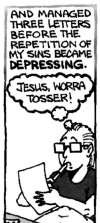

WITHIN DAYS, SYMPTOMS OF THE BIG C CAME RUSHING BACK.

YOU OKAY, LUV?

OH, FINE.

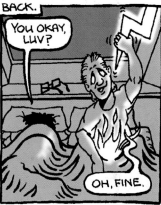

THEN WE ENTERTAINED OUR FIRST HOUSE-GUESTS, **SKUNK** AND **SAM**, A COUPLE OF BIKERS FROM DARKEST LINCOLNSHIRE, JUDY'S HOME COUNTY.

GROWL

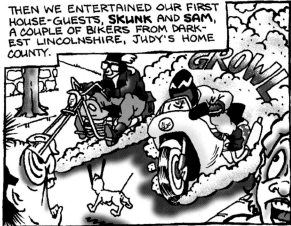

GET KETTLE ON.

I'VE GOT THE CUPCAKES!

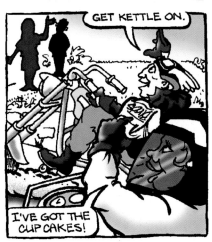

THE STREET WAS SUDDENLY CLEARED OF WIVES, DAUGHTERS AND **DOGS**.

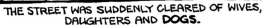

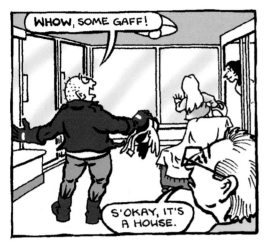

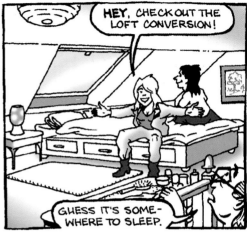

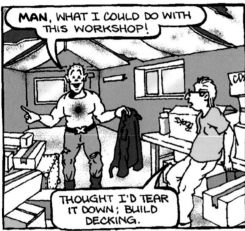

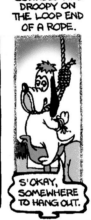

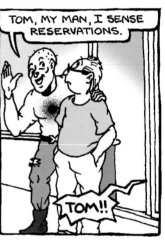

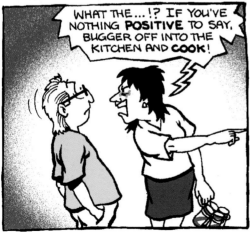

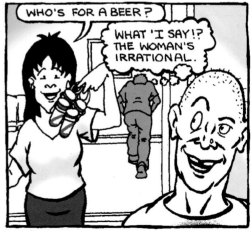

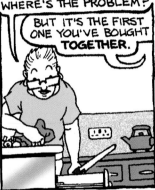

IT'S A **HOUSE**, F'CHRISS-AKE; FOUR WALLS AND A LIFETIME OF DEBT. WHERE'S THE PROBLEM?

BUT IT'S THE FIRST ONE YOU'VE BOUGHT **TOGETHER**.

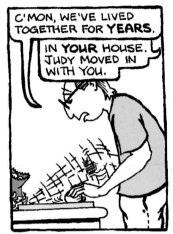

C'MON, WE'VE LIVED TOGETHER FOR **YEARS**.

IN **YOUR** HOUSE. JUDY MOVED IN WITH YOU.

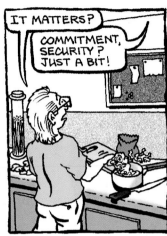

IT MATTERS?

COMMITMENT, SECURITY? JUST A BIT!

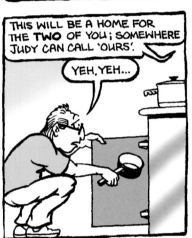

THIS WILL BE A HOME FOR THE **TWO** OF YOU; SOMEWHERE JUDY CAN CALL 'OURS'.

YEH, YEH...

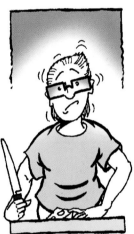

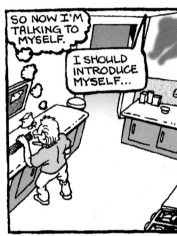

SO NOW I'M TALKING TO MYSELF.

I SHOULD INTRODUCE MYSELF...

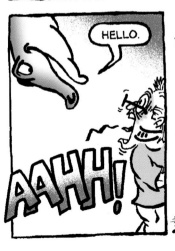

HELLO.

AAHH!

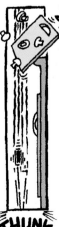

THUNK

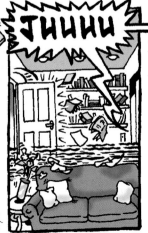

JUUUU—

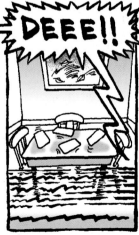

DEEE!!

35

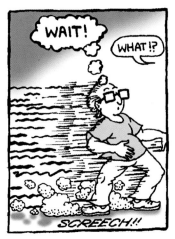

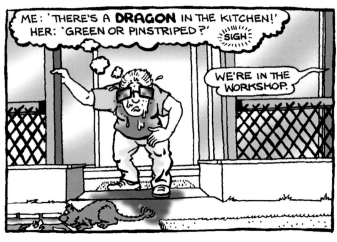

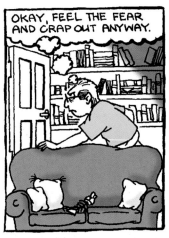

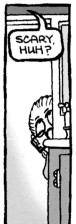

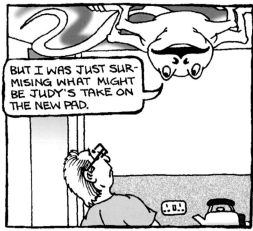

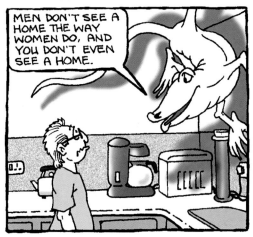

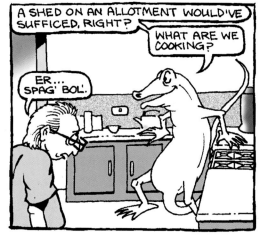

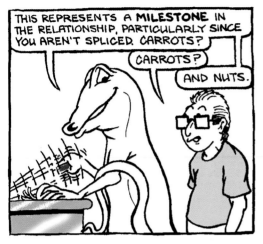

THIS REPRESENTS A **MILESTONE** IN THE RELATIONSHIP, PARTICULARLY SINCE YOU AREN'T SPLICED. CARROTS?

CARROTS?

AND NUTS.

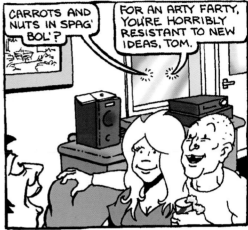

CARROTS AND NUTS IN SPAG' BOL'?

FOR AN ARTY FARTY, YOU'RE HORRIBLY RESISTANT TO NEW IDEAS, TOM.

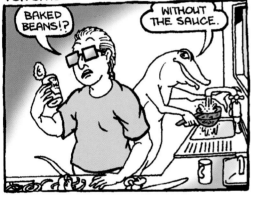

I HADN'T A CLUE WHERE HE SPRANG FROM OR WHERE HE GOT HIS RECIPE FOR SPAGHETTI BOLOGNESE...

BAKED BEANS!?

WITHOUT THE SAUCE.

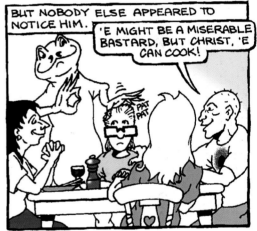

BUT NOBODY ELSE APPEARED TO NOTICE HIM.

'E MIGHT BE A MISERABLE BASTARD, BUT CHRIST, 'E CAN COOK!

PAT PAT

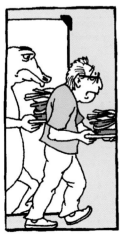

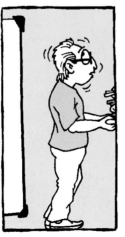

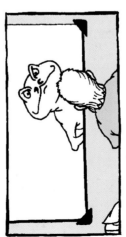

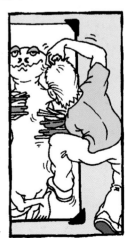

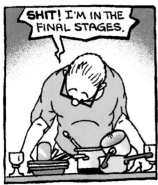

SHIT! I'M IN THE FINAL STAGES.

THE HALLUCINATION WAS CLEAR EVIDENCE MY CONDITION HAD RADICALLY DETERIORATED.

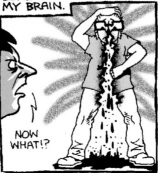

IN LESS THAN THREE MONTHS, THE CANCER HAD SURREPTITIOUSLY GNAWED ITS WAY UP MY BACKBONE AND STARTED IN ON MY BRAIN.

NOW WHAT!?

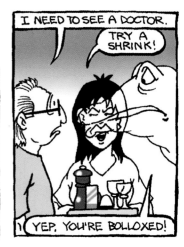

I NEED TO SEE A DOCTOR.

TRY A SHRINK!

YEP, YOU'RE BOLLOXED!

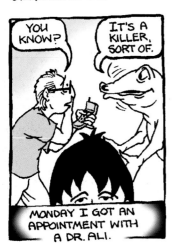

YOU KNOW?

IT'S A KILLER, SORT OF.

MONDAY I GOT AN APPOINTMENT WITH A DR. ALI.

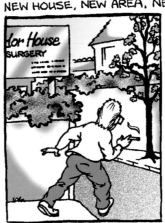

NEW HOUSE, NEW AREA, NEW SURGERY, NEW DOCTOR...

dor House SURGERY

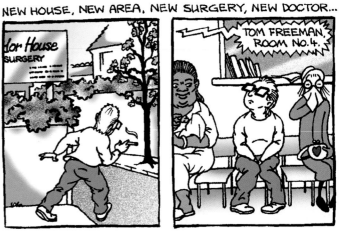

TOM FREEMAN, ROOM NO. 4.

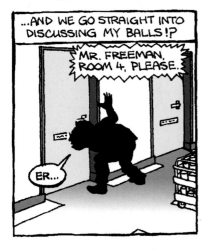

...AND WE GO STRAIGHT INTO DISCUSSING MY BALLS!?

MR. FREEMAN, ROOM 4, PLEASE..

ER...

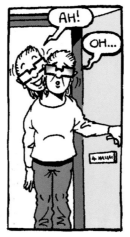

AH!

OH...

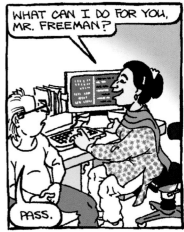

WHAT CAN I DO FOR YOU, MR. FREEMAN?

PASS.

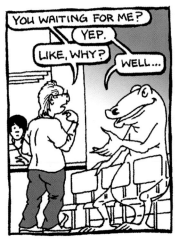

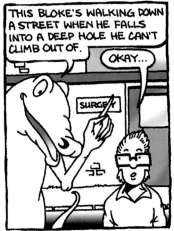

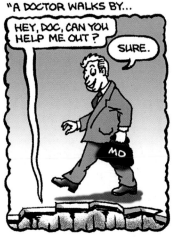

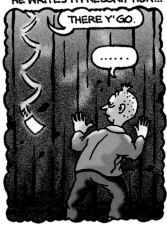

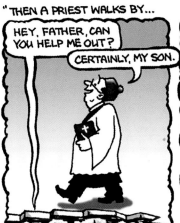

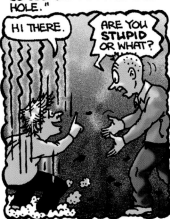

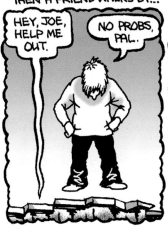

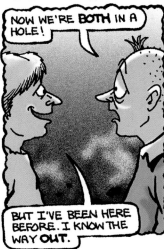

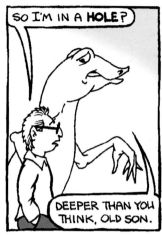

SO I'M IN A **HOLE**?

DEEPER THAN YOU THINK, OLD SON.

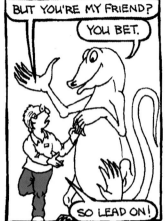

BUT YOU'RE MY FRIEND?

YOU BET.

SO LEAD ON!

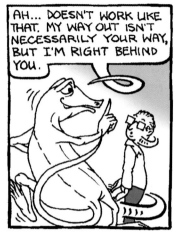

AH... DOESN'T WORK LIKE THAT. MY WAY OUT ISN'T NECESSARILY YOUR WAY, BUT I'M RIGHT BEHIND YOU.

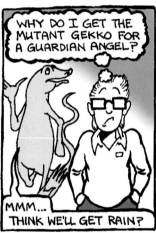

WHY DO I GET THE MUTANT GEKKO FOR A GUARDIAN ANGEL?

MMM... THINK WE'LL GET RAIN?

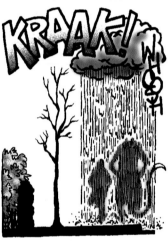

KRAAK!

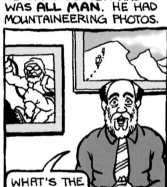

TWO DAYS LATER I GOT TO SEE A DOCTOR WHO WAS **ALL MAN**. HE HAD MOUNTAINEERING PHOTOS.

WHAT'S THE PROBLEM?

IN A MATTER-OF-FACT MANNER (AS MUCH AS TO SAY, "I'M WAY AHEAD OF YOU ON THIS!"), I LISTED THE SYMPTOMS OF MY CANCER.

HMM... **NASTY.**

I WAS COOL. MY AFFAIRS WERE IN ORDER. HOWEVER LONG I HAD - YEARS, MONTHS, WEEKS - I HAD A LIST OF 'THINGS TO DO BEFORE I DIE'. SETTLING MY TAX BILL DIDN'T FEATURE. LOTS OF DEVIANT SEX DID.

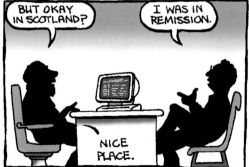

BUT OKAY IN SCOTLAND?

I WAS IN REMISSION.

NICE PLACE.

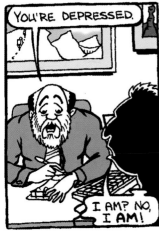

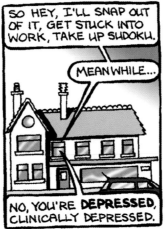

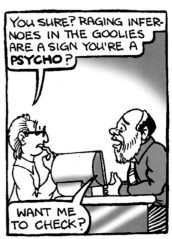

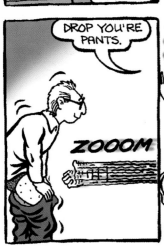

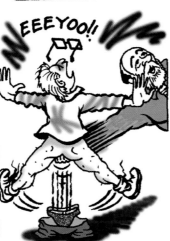

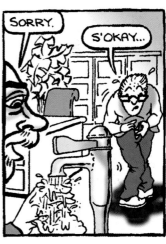

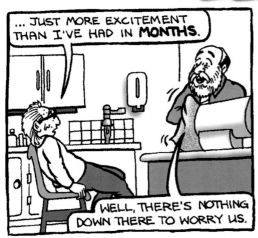

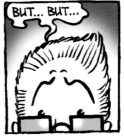

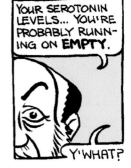

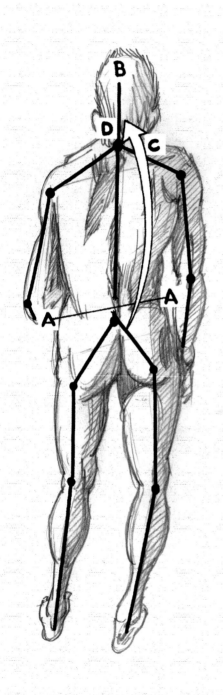

The way Dr. Matterhorn explained it, serotonin is the juice that controls our **MOODS**. When we are running on empty, weird shit happens in the body.

Somewhere around 'A', a logjam appears, blocking the flow of information from **SOUTH** of the dam to the very **NORTH** – the brain ('B').

So the south musters an army of navvies to build a channel ('C') straight to the brain, by-passing all the neuro canals, locks and junctions of the north, south of the neck ('D').

Unimpeded, the channel spirits great bores of information to headquarters. Drowning in all this exclusive and apparently **CRUCIAL** intelligence, the brain is prone to misdiagnose a stubbed toe as cause for immediate amputation of **BOTH LEGS**!

Whatever was going on with my bollocks, the greatly exaggerated message, rushed through to H.Q. caused **MELTDOWN**.

I was **DYING**.

FORCE QUIT was imminent!

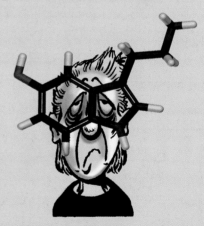

According to the doc, the remedy lay in a type of pill known as an **SSRI**, a 'selective serotonin re-uptake inhibitor'.

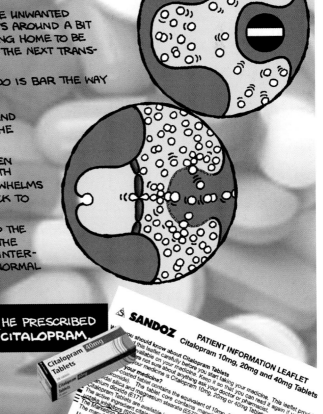

Somewhere in command H.Q., a neuro-transmitter ('X') is pumping out a steady stream of serotonin ('Y') in the firm belief it is being picked up by an active receiver ('Z').

Unfortunately, the receiver is DOWN. Convinced it has all the serotonin it can handle, it has automatically shut off.

In fact the stores are EMPTY and the receiver is malfunctioning.

Meanwhile, the unwanted serotonin wafts around a bit before returning home to be stored pending the next transmission.

What SSRIs do is bar the way home.

The pills build a BOOM round the transmitter that lets the juice out but not back in.

Over time, the gap between 'X' and 'Z' becomes stiff with serotonin that finally overwhelms the receiver, forcing it back to work.

Six months on, it is hoped the receiver has rediscovered the benefits of taking in an uninterrupted flow of juice, and normal service is resumed.

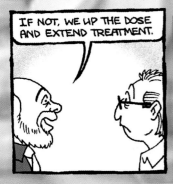

IF NOT, WE UP THE DOSE AND EXTEND TREATMENT.

HE PRESCRIBED CITALOPRAM.

Citalopram 40mg
Tablets

43

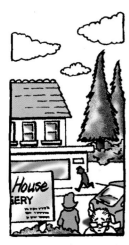

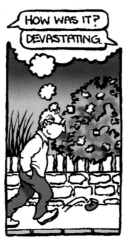

HOW WAS IT?
DEVASTATING.

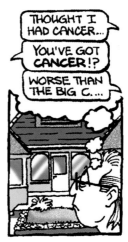

THOUGHT I HAD CANCER...
YOU'VE GOT CANCER!?
WORSE THAN THE BIG C....

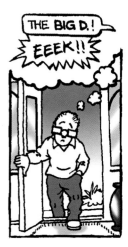

THE BIG D.!
EEEK!!

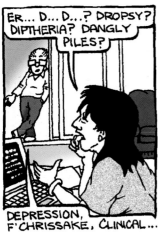

ER... D...D...? DROPSY? DIPTHERIA? DANGLY PILES?

DEPRESSION, F'CHRISSAKE, CLINICAL...

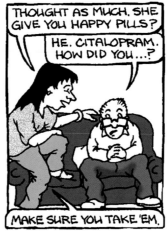

THOUGHT AS MUCH. SHE GIVE YOU HAPPY PILLS?
HE. CITALOPRAM. HOW DID YOU...?

MAKE SURE YOU TAKE 'EM.

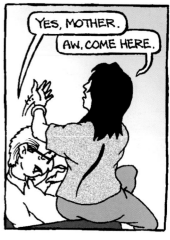

YES, MOTHER.
AW, COME HERE.

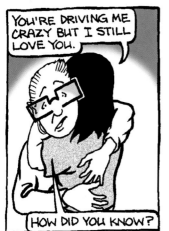

YOU'RE DRIVING ME CRAZY BUT I STILL LOVE YOU.

HOW DID YOU KNOW?

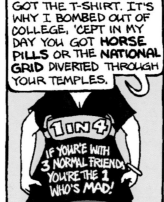

GOT THE T-SHIRT. IT'S WHY I BOMBED OUT OF COLLEGE, 'CEPT IN MY DAY YOU GOT HORSE PILLS OR THE NATIONAL GRID DIVERTED THROUGH YOUR TEMPLES.

1 IN 4
IF YOU'RE WITH 3 NORMAL FRIENDS YOU'RE THE 1 WHO'S MAD!

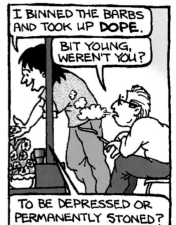

I BINNED THE BARBS AND TOOK UP DOPE.
BIT YOUNG, WEREN'T YOU?

TO BE DEPRESSED OR PERMANENTLY STONED?

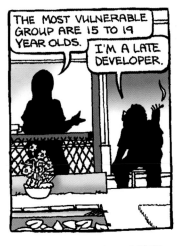

THE MOST VULNERABLE GROUP ARE 15 TO 19 YEAR OLDS.

I'M A LATE DEVELOPER.

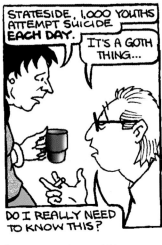

STATESIDE, 1,000 YOUTHS ATTEMPT SUICIDE **EACH DAY.**

IT'S A GOTH THING...

DO I REALLY NEED TO KNOW THIS?

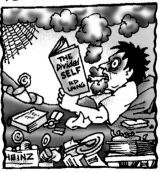

"DEPENDS. I BECAME **OBSESSED.** READ EVERYTHING GOING ON MADNESS. DIDN'T GET OUT OF BED FOR **TWO MONTHS.**

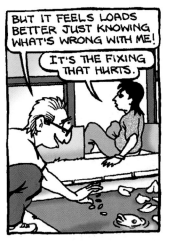

"I LIVED ON COLD CREAMED RICE AND SIX-SKINNERS. THE PLACE **STANK.** DROVE MY FLATMATES TO DESPAIR.

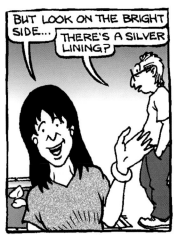

"TOOK ME FOUR MONTHS TO SIGN ON SICK, SIX BEFORE I COULD FACE TOWN. YOU'RE IN FOR A BAD TIME."

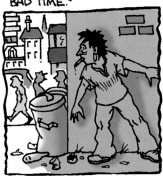

BUT IT FEELS LOADS BETTER JUST KNOWING WHAT'S WRONG WITH ME!

IT'S THE FIXING THAT HURTS.

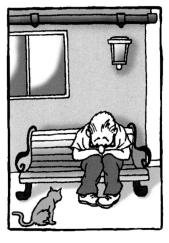

BUT LOOK ON THE BRIGHT SIDE...

THERE'S A SILVER LINING?

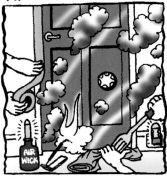

AT LAST WE'VE GOT **SOMETHING IN COMMON!**

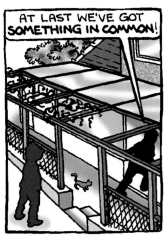

IF ANYTHING, JUDY AND I HAVE TOO MUCH IN COMMON, POSSIBLY EXPLAINING WHY OUR SPATS MADE BASRA LOOK LIKE **CLUB MED.**

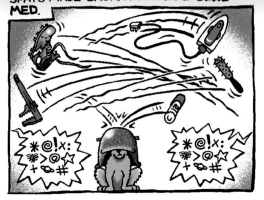

WE BOTH WORK AT HOME, ME ON **CHALK**, HER ON **CHEESE** (SHE MAKES CORSAGES, WHICH SELL FOR SILLY SUMS ON EBAY).

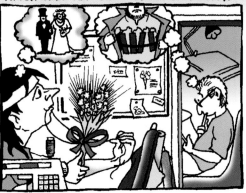

WE BOTH LOVE EXPLORING THE GREAT OUTDOORS, HER LOWLANDS, ME HIGH.

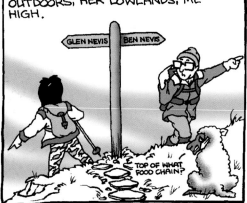

WE ARE BOTH STRONG-WILLED, COMPETITIVE **MARD ARSES**, BARELY SUFFERING EACH OTHER'S TASTE IN MUSIC, FILMS AND CRAP TV.

DESPERATE HOUSEWIVES!

HEROES!

AND WE EACH HARBOURED A DEEP SEATED **ANGER**, HER FOR HER VIOLENT, ALCOHOLIC FATHER (RIP), ME FOR... I WASN'T SURE!

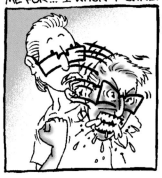

WE HAD BEEN TOGETHER A DECADE AND MORE, SHARED SOME TIMES OF OUR LIVES, AND TOO OFTEN BEEN TWO DIVORCE LAWYERS SHY OF BUSTING UP.

IT WAS A MATCH MADE IN **HELL** (LINCOLNSHIRE), BUT REALISING I HAD MADE THE PAST YEAR PURGATORY FOR JUDY WAS A BLACKER CORNER OF HADES.

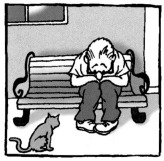

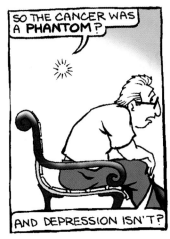

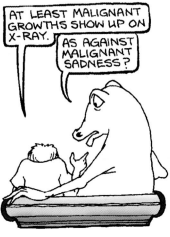

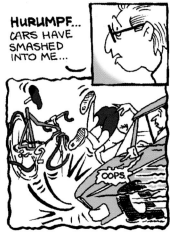

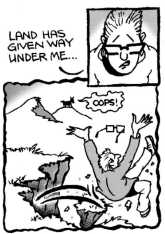

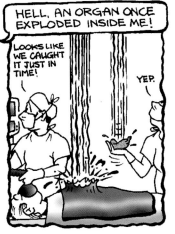

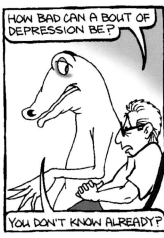

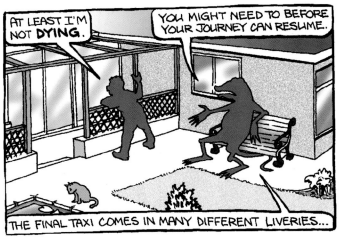

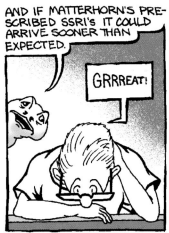

47

FUNNY THING ABOUT WHITE MAN'S MEDICINE; THEY DIAGNOSE A PSYCHOLOGICAL DISORDER THEN GO TO WORK ON YOUR **CHEMISTRY**.

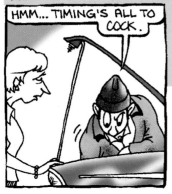

HMM... TIMING'S ALL TO COCK.

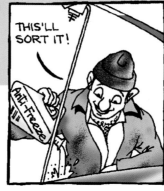

THIS'LL SORT IT!

Anti-Freeze

PROBLEM IS, THEY DON'T KNOW AS MUCH ABOUT THE CHEMISTRY OF THE BRAIN AS DRUG COMPANIES LIKE TO BELIEVE. SEROTONIN IS ALSO THOUGHT TO IMPACT ON OUR BIOLOGICAL THERMOSTAT, SENSORY PERCEPTIONS AND SLEEP PATTERNS, BUT **WHAT ELSE**?

SO WHAT IF I TOOK THE ODD SEROXAT WHILE I WAS PREGNANT?

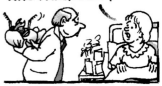

INDEPENDENT TESTS ON THE SIX MOST POPULAR SSRIS DISCOVERED THAT, IN 80% OF CASES, THEY WERE NO MORE EFFECTIVE THAN A PLACEBO (SUGAR PILL).

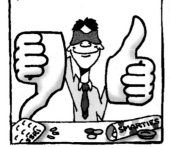

SMARTIES

AT THE SAME TIME, THE DRUG COMPANIES FREELY ADMIT HAPPY PILLS CAN HAVE UP TO **300** SIDE EFFECTS, THOUGH MINOR REACTIONS LIKE BIRTH DEFECTS AND HEIGHTENED VULNERABILITY TO SUICIDE DON'T MAKE THE SMALL PRINT.

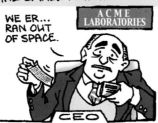

WE ER... RAN OUT OF SPACE.

ACME LABORATORIES

CEO

FOR SOME, A QUIET MELANCHOLIA CAN MUTATE INTO HOMICIDAL RAGE AT THE DROP OF AN SSRI.

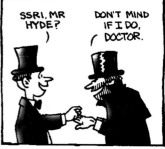

SSRI, MR HYDE?

DON'T MIND IF I DO, DOCTOR.

AND WHY GO LOOKING FOR A VICTIM WHEN THE MAN IN THE MIRROR IS JUST ASKING TO BE WHACKED?

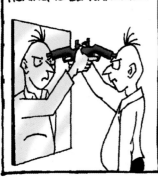

THE UK SPENDS OVER £**420M** A YEAR ON 'ANTI-DEPRESSANTS', AND SIX MILLION OF US REACH FOR THEM MORNING, NOON OR NIGHT.

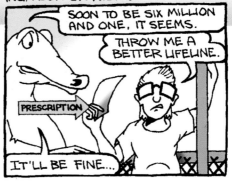

SOON TO BE SIX MILLION AND ONE, IT SEEMS.

THROW ME A BETTER LIFELINE.

PRESCRIPTION

IT'LL BE FINE...

CITALOPRAM ONLY HAS 113 SIDE EFFECTS!

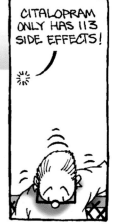

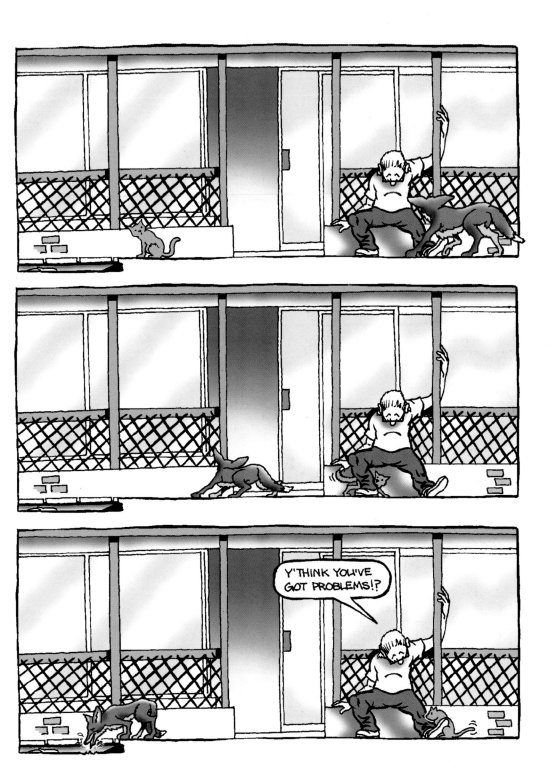

49

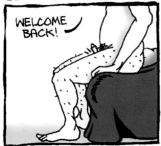
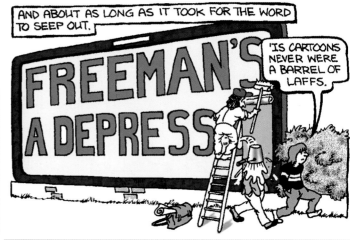
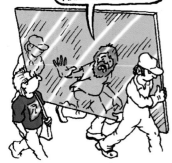
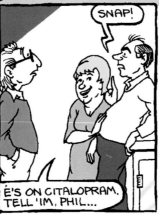
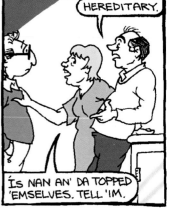
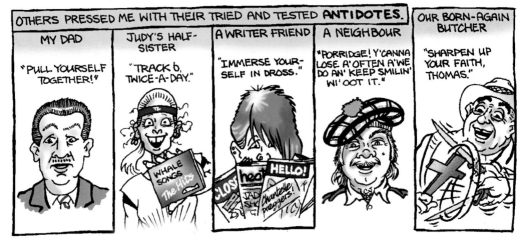

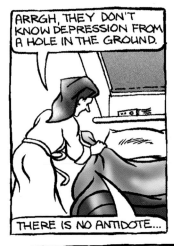

ARRGH, THEY DON'T KNOW DEPRESSION FROM A HOLE IN THE GROUND.

THERE IS NO ANTIDOTE...

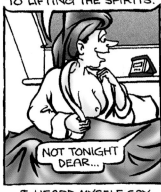

BUT I FOUND A GOOD SHAG WENT A LONG WAY TO LIFTING THE SPIRITS.

NOT TONIGHT DEAR...

...I HEARD MYSELF SAY.

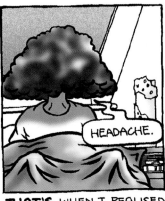

HEADACHE.

THAT'S WHEN I REALISED THE **GRAVITY** OF MY ILLNESS.

THAT AND A HUMILIATING ATTEMPT AT THE 'ARE WE NOT **MEN**?' APPROACH TO ADVERSITY. I HURLED MYSELF HEADLONG INTO **WORK**.

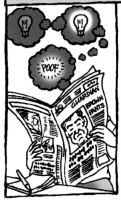

POOF

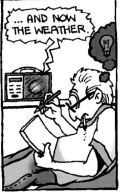

... AND NOW THE WEATHER.

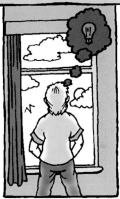

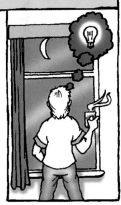

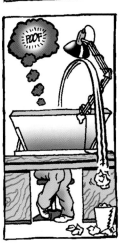

POOF

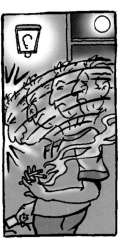

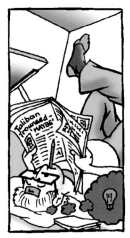

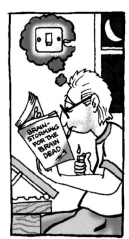

51

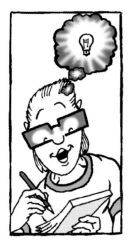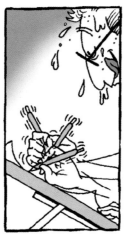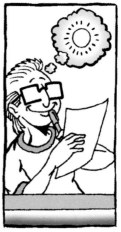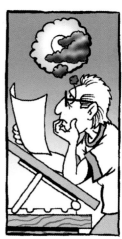

I COULD HAVE DECORATED THE BUNGALOW, TWO COATS, IN THE TIME IT TOOK ME TO WHIP UP THIS LITTLE RIB-TICKLER...

YEP, WELL AND TRULY **BOLLOXED**!

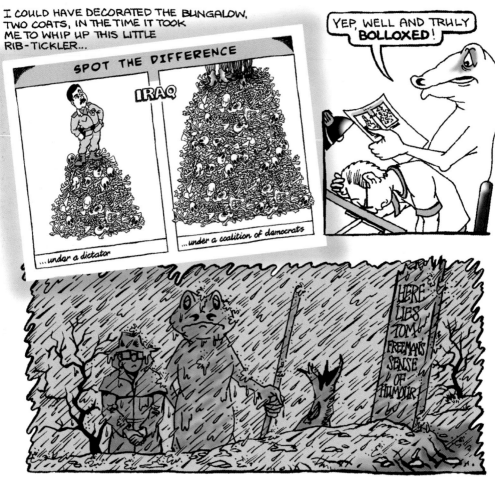

SPOT THE DIFFERENCE

IRAQ

...under a dictator

...under a coalition of democrats

HERE LIES TOM FREEMAN'S SENSE OF HUMOUR

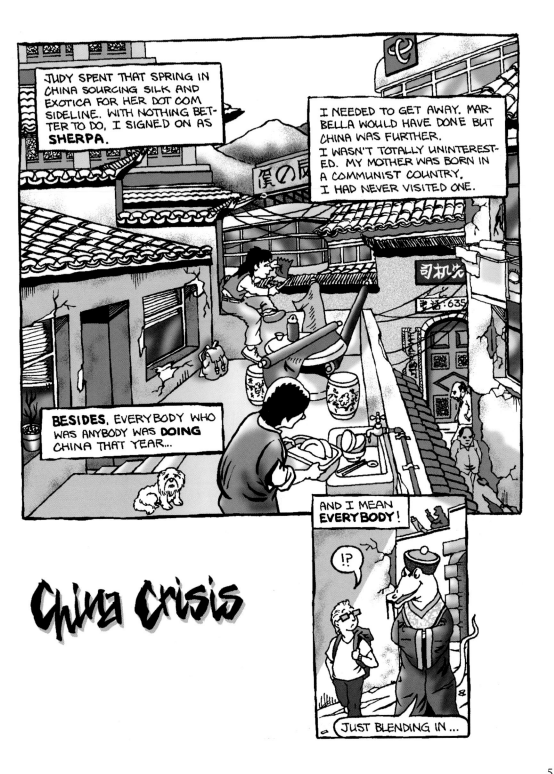

JUDY SPENT THAT SPRING IN CHINA SOURCING SILK AND EXOTICA FOR HER DOT COM SIDELINE. WITH NOTHING BETTER TO DO, I SIGNED ON AS **SHERPA**.

I NEEDED TO GET AWAY. MARBELLA WOULD HAVE DONE BUT CHINA WAS FURTHER.
I WASN'T TOTALLY UNINTERESTED. MY MOTHER WAS BORN IN A COMMUNIST COUNTRY, I HAD NEVER VISITED ONE.

BESIDES, EVERYBODY WHO WAS ANYBODY WAS **DOING** CHINA THAT YEAR...

AND I MEAN **EVERYBODY**!

!?

_ JUST BLENDING IN ...

China Crisis

WHILE THE HORDES OF WESTERN TOURISTS BURNED A YETI-SIZE CARBON FOOTPRINT JETTING BETWEEN PHOTO-SHOOTS ...

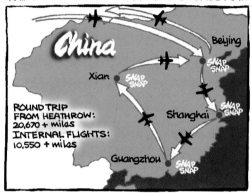

AND THE MEDIA SCOURED COASTAL CITIES FOR STORIES THAT REINFORCED OUR PREJUDICES ABOUT 'INSCRUTABLE' OR 'INHUMANE' ORIENTALS, ...

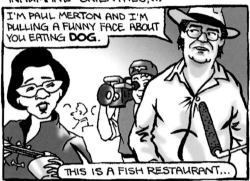

I'M PAUL MERTON AND I'M PULLING A FUNNY FACE ABOUT YOU EATING **DOG**.

THIS IS A FISH RESTAURANT...

WE FOUND OURSELVES IN A SMALL TOWN IN HUBEI PROVINCE WHERE WHITES WERE SO RARE WE CAUSED **ACCIDENTS**.

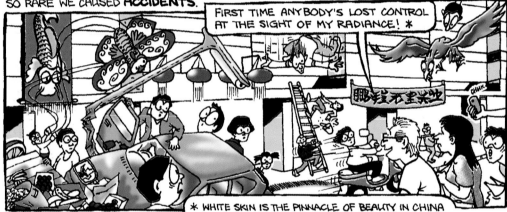

FIRST TIME ANYBODY'S LOST CONTROL AT THE SIGHT OF MY RADIANCE! *

* WHITE SKIN IS THE PINNACLE OF BEAUTY IN CHINA

EATING OUT, WE TOOK OUR LIVES INTO OUR HANDS AS SALVOS OF INVITATIONS TO DRINK A TOAST AT THEIR TABLE RAINED IN LIKE **FRIENDLY FIRE.**

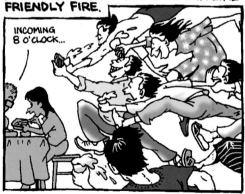

INCOMING 8 O'CLOCK...

THE GENEROSITY OF OUR HOSTS WAS EMBARRASSING. HOW MANY **FEASTS** CAN A WESTERN STOMACH TAKE WEEK AFTER WEEK!?

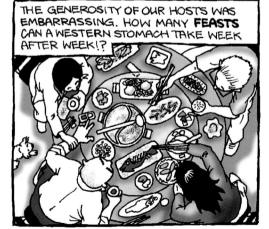

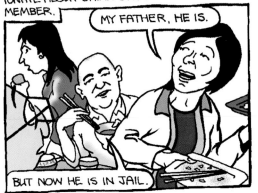

NUYING WAS CHIEF RESEARCHER AT THE JIANGLING SILK INSTITUTE. SHE WAS PASSIONATE ABOUT CHINA BUT NOT A PARTY MEMBER.

MY FATHER, HE IS.

BUT NOW HE IS IN JAIL.

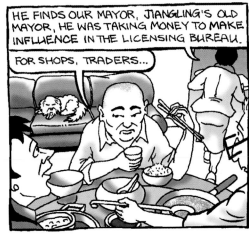

HE FINDS OUR MAYOR, JIANGLING'S OLD MAYOR, HE WAS TAKING MONEY TO MAKE INFLUENCE IN THE LICENSING BUREAU.

FOR SHOPS, TRADERS...

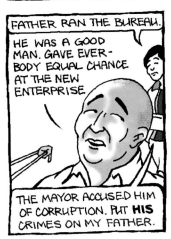

FATHER RAN THE BUREAU.

HE WAS A GOOD MAN. GAVE EVERYBODY EQUAL CHANCE AT THE NEW ENTERPRISE.

THE MAYOR ACCUSED HIM OF CORRUPTION. PUT **HIS** CRIMES ON MY FATHER.

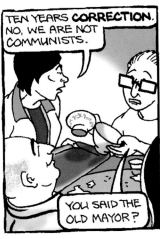

TEN YEARS **CORRECTION**. NO, WE ARE NOT COMMUNISTS.

YOU SAID THE OLD MAYOR?

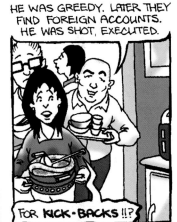

HE WAS GREEDY. LATER THEY FIND FOREIGN ACCOUNTS. HE WAS SHOT, EXECUTED.

FOR **KICK-BACKS** !!?

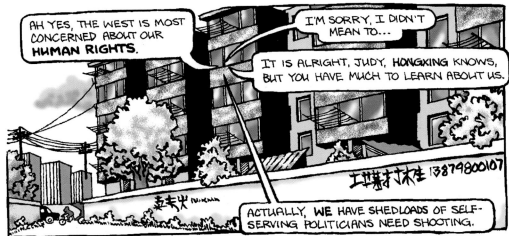

AH YES, THE WEST IS MOST CONCERNED ABOUT OUR **HUMAN RIGHTS**.

I'M SORRY, I DIDN'T MEAN TO...

IT IS ALRIGHT, JUDY, **HONGXING** KNOWS, BUT YOU HAVE MUCH TO LEARN ABOUT US.

ACTUALLY, **WE** HAVE SHEDLOADS OF SELF-SERVING POLITICIANS NEED SHOOTING.

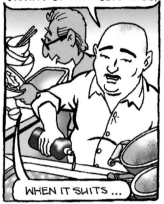

HUMAN RIGHTS ARE THE WORRY OF RICH COUNTRIES.

WHEN IT SUITS ...

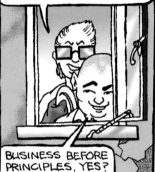

BUT FIND A CHINESE SWEAT SHOP THAT CAN KNOCK OUT BLUE JEANS CHEAPER THAN A MEXICAN...

BUSINESS BEFORE PRINCIPLES, YES?

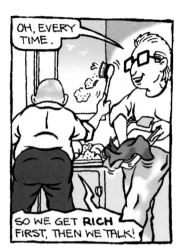

OH, EVERY TIME.

SO WE GET **RICH** FIRST, THEN WE TALK!

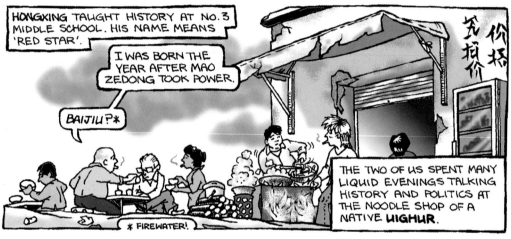

HONGXING TAUGHT HISTORY AT NO. 3 MIDDLE SCHOOL. HIS NAME MEANS 'RED STAR'.

I WAS BORN THE YEAR AFTER MAO ZEDONG TOOK POWER.

BAIJIU?*

* FIREWATER!

THE TWO OF US SPENT MANY LIQUID EVENINGS TALKING HISTORY AND POLITICS AT THE NOODLE SHOP OF A NATIVE **UIGHUR**.

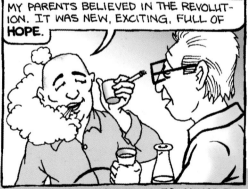

MY PARENTS BELIEVED IN THE REVOLUTION. IT WAS NEW, EXCITING, FULL OF **HOPE**.

UIGHURS ARE A DISTRUSTED MINORITY. WALLS DO NOT HAVE EARS IN A UIGHUR SHOP.

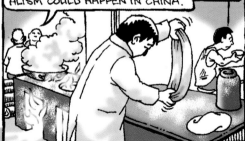

EVEN THROUGH THE FAMINE AND THE MADNESS OF THE CULTURAL REVOLUTION, THEY BELIEVED SOMETHING BETTER THAN FEUDALISM COULD HAPPEN IN CHINA.

THAT SAID, I WAS SURPRISED HOW OPENLY STRANGERS DISCUSSED CHINA'S FUTURE WITH ME.

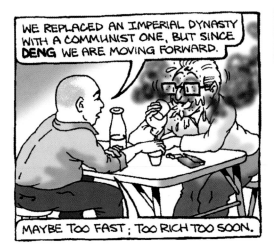

WE REPLACED AN IMPERIAL DYNASTY WITH A COMMUNIST ONE, BUT SINCE **DENG** WE ARE MOVING FORWARD.

MAYBE TOO FAST; TOO RICH TOO SOON.

DENG XIAOPING WAS **HONGXING'S** HERO, A PRAGMATIST WHO ACTUALLY DID COME FROM PEASANT STOCK AND NEVER FORGOT IT.

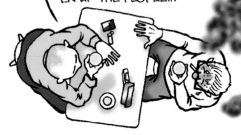

IMAGINE YOU WERE BORN IN A LAND WHERE NO INDUSTRIAL REVOLUTION, NO RENAISSANCE OR ENLIGHTENMENT HAS SHAKEN UP THE PEOPLE...

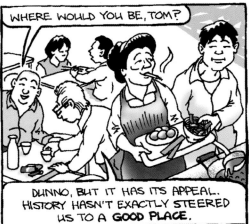

WHERE WOULD YOU BE, TOM?

DUNNO, BUT IT HAS ITS APPEAL. HISTORY HASN'T EXACTLY STEERED US TO A **GOOD PLACE.**

WE HAVE NO HISTORY, ONLY A LONG LONG PAST OF ONE DYNASTY AFTER ANOTHER. HAN, MONGUL, MANCHU... NO DIFFERENT FOR THE PEOPLE.

THE COMMUNISTS?

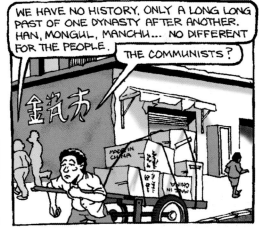

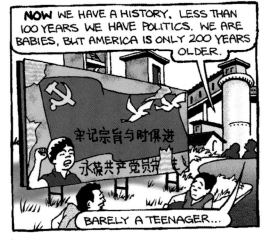

NOW WE HAVE A HISTORY, LESS THAN 100 YEARS WE HAVE POLITICS. WE ARE BABIES, BUT AMERICA IS ONLY 200 YEARS OLDER.

BARELY A TEENAGER...

AND SUCH A MODEL OF DEMOCRACY!!

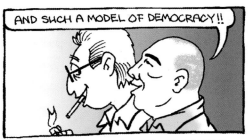

IRONY IS NOT A FEATURE OF CHINESE HUMOUR AND SATIRE BARELY REGISTERS. NUYING AND **HONGXING** HAD WORKED ABROAD IN COMMUNIST COUNTRIES THAT RUBBED SHOULDERS WITH THE WEST. THEY HAD SEEN OUR TV. RADIO FREE EUROPE AND THE WORLD SERVICE TAUGHT THEM ENGLISH.

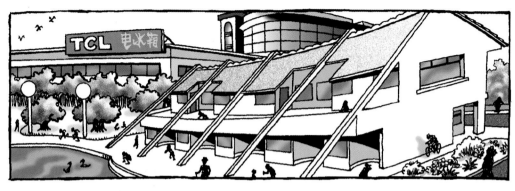

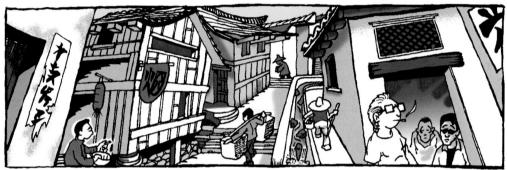

MUCH OF MY TIME IN JIANGLING WAS SPENT WALKING THE STREETS, SOAKING UP THE BUZZ OF A SMALL TOWN IN THE THROES OF BIG CHANGES.

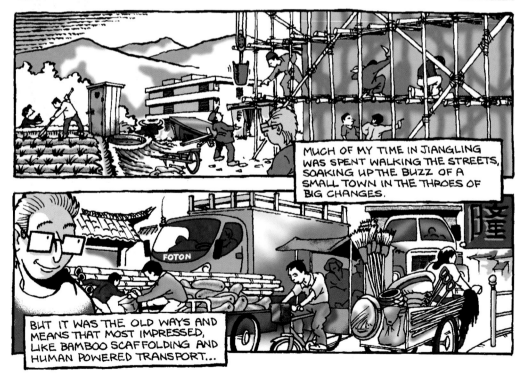

BUT IT WAS THE OLD WAYS AND MEANS THAT MOST IMPRESSED, LIKE BAMBOO SCAFFOLDING AND HUMAN POWERED TRANSPORT...

LIKE OBSESSIVE RECYCLING THAT PUT THE WEST TO SHAME...

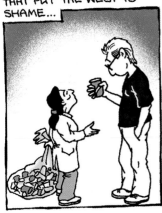

BOUNTIFUL DOWNTOWN SMALL HOLDINGS, 100% ORGANIC...

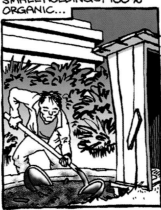

DAILY STREET SWEEPING, WEEKLY FURNITURE POLISHING...

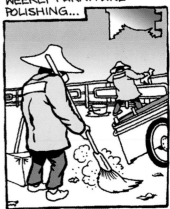

AND THE ENERGY OF PEOPLE! EVERY STREET WAS AT THE SAME TIME A HIVE OF INDUSTRY AND THROBBING SOCIAL CLUB.

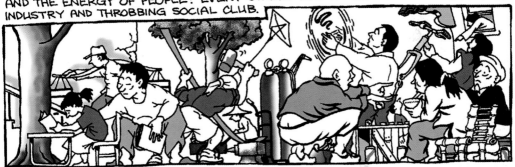

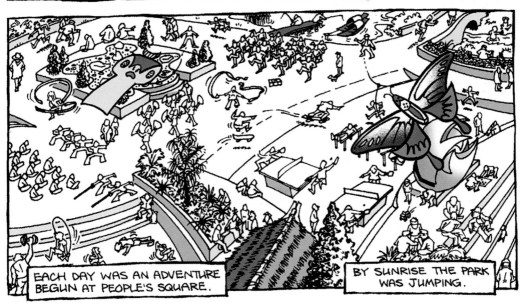

EACH DAY WAS AN ADVENTURE BEGUN AT PEOPLE'S SQUARE.

BY SUNRISE THE PARK WAS JUMPING.

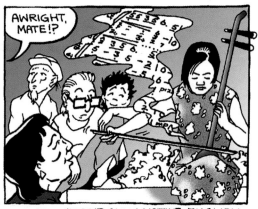

AWRIGHT, MATE!?

WE WEREN'T THE ONLY NATIVE ENGLISH SPEAKERS IN TOWN.

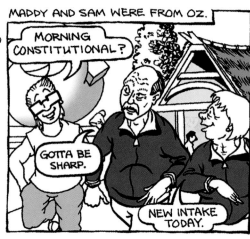

MADDY AND SAM WERE FROM OZ.

MORNING CONSTITUTIONAL?

GOTTA BE SHARP.

NEW INTAKE TODAY.

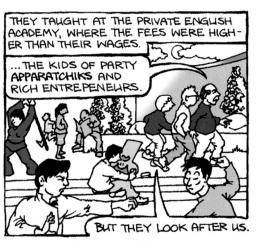

THEY TAUGHT AT THE PRIVATE ENGLISH ACADEMY, WHERE THE FEES WERE HIGHER THAN THEIR WAGES.

...THE KIDS OF PARTY **APPARATCHIKS** AND RICH ENTREPENEURS.

BUT THEY LOOK AFTER US.

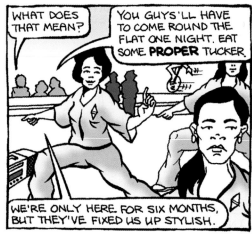

WHAT DOES THAT MEAN?

YOU GUYS'LL HAVE TO COME ROUND THE FLAT ONE NIGHT. EAT SOME **PROPER** TUCKER.

WE'RE ONLY HERE FOR SIX MONTHS, BUT THEY'VE FIXED US UP STYLISH.

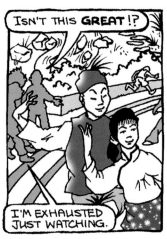

ISN'T THIS **GREAT**!?

I'M EXHAUSTED JUST WATCHING.

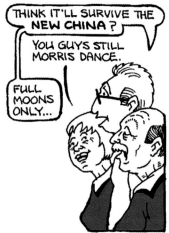

THINK IT'LL SURVIVE THE **NEW CHINA**?

YOU GUYS STILL MORRIS DANCE.

FULL MOONS ONLY...

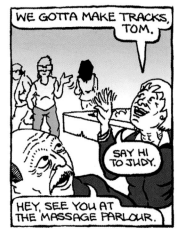

WE GOTTA MAKE TRACKS, TOM.

SAY HI TO JUDY.

HEY, SEE YOU AT THE MASSAGE PARLOUR.

THAT JUNE SEVERAL SATELLITE VILLAGES FAILED TO ENTER THEIR DRAGON BOATS IN THE DUANWU JIE FESTIVAL. NO MEN. ALL HAD LEFT TO SEEK WORK IN THE CITIES.

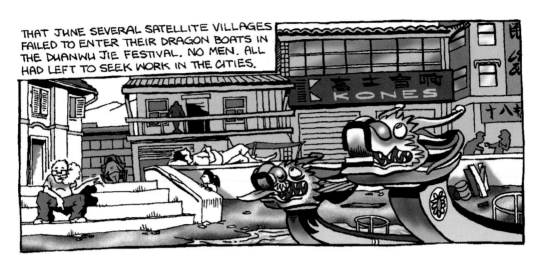

A 2,000 YEAR OLD TRADITION DIDN'T JUST FIZZLE OUT. IT **DROPPED DEAD**. CHINA WAS SPRINTING FULL PELT INTO A SHIT LOAD OF TROUBLE.

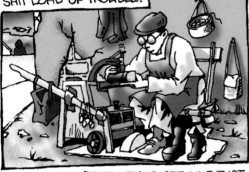

INDUSTRIAL REVOLUTIONS ARE LIKE THAT.

HONGXING LAUGHED WHEN I EXPLAINED THE EXPRESSION, 'SHIT'S GONNA HIT THE FAN'.

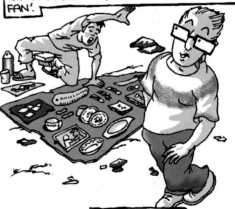

I ASKED HIM TO WRITE IT IN CHINESE. HE SAID HE COULDN'T. THE LANGUAGE DIDN'T ALLOW FOR ANYTHING IN THE FUTURE TO BE SO UNEQUIVOCALLY **NEGATIVE**.

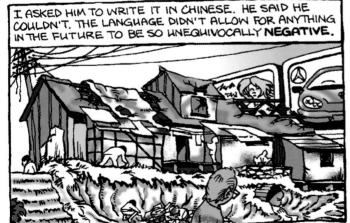

I **LIKED** THAT.

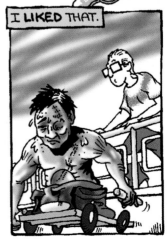

61

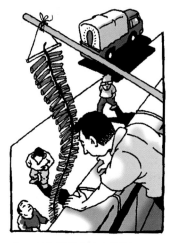

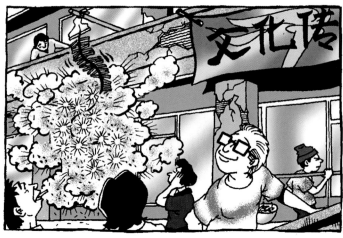

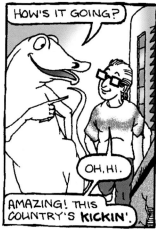

HOW'S IT GOING?

OH, HI.

AMAZING! THIS COUNTRY'S **KICKIN'**.

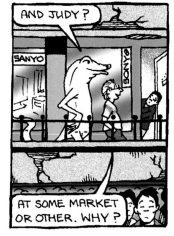

AND JUDY?

AT SOME MARKET OR OTHER. WHY?

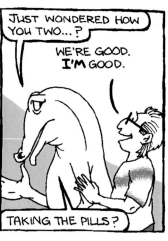

JUST WONDERED HOW YOU TWO...?

WE'RE GOOD. **I'M** GOOD.

TAKING THE PILLS?

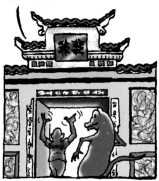

KEEP FORGETTING, BUT THE EXCITEMENT OF THIS PLACE... I'M **GUSHING** SEROTONIN!

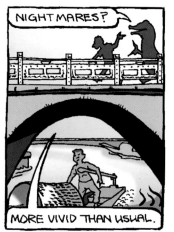

NIGHTMARES?

MORE VIVID THAN USUAL.

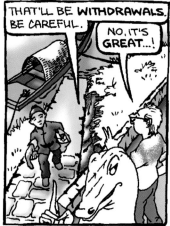

THAT'LL BE **WITHDRAWALS**. BE CAREFUL.

NO, IT'S GREAT...!

"HORRIFIC THINGS NOW APPEAR IN GROOVY LOCATIONS RATHER THAN GREYSVILLE."

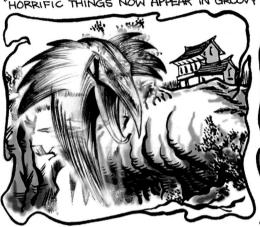

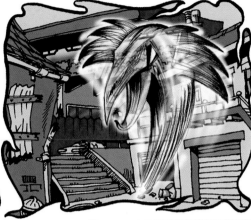

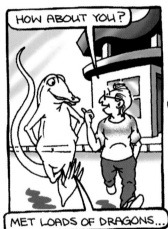

HOW ABOUT YOU?

MET LOADS OF DRAGONS...

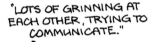
"LOTS OF GRINNING AT EACH OTHER, TRYING TO COMMUNICATE."

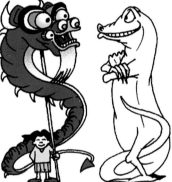

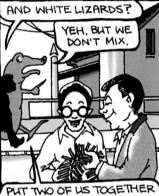

AND WHITE LIZARDS?

YEH, BUT WE DON'T MIX.

PUT TWO OF US TOGETHER AND SOME POOR SAP'S GONNA CATCH ST. PETER NAPPING.

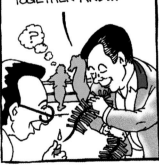

BACK HOME, NOBODY SEEMS BOTHERED. IN CHINA, THE VAGUEST HINT OF US GETTING TOGETHER AND...

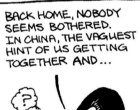

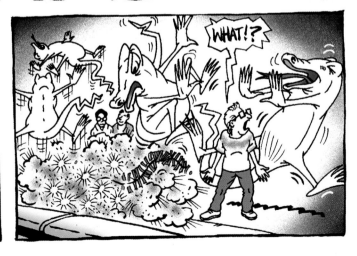

WHAT!?

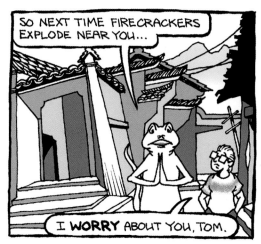

SO NEXT TIME FIRECRACKERS EXPLODE NEAR YOU...

I **WORRY** ABOUT YOU, TOM.

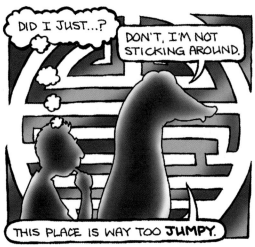

DID I JUST...?

DON'T, I'M NOT STICKING AROUND.

THIS PLACE IS WAY TOO **JUMPY**.

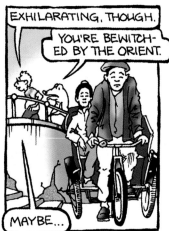

EXHILARATING, THOUGH.

YOU'RE BEWITCHED BY THE ORIENT.

MAYBE...

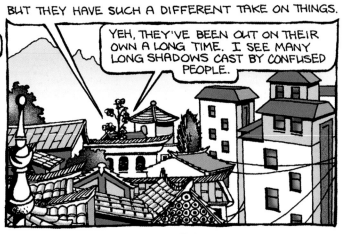

BUT THEY HAVE SUCH A DIFFERENT TAKE ON THINGS.

YEH, THEY'VE BEEN OUT ON THEIR OWN A LONG TIME. I SEE MANY LONG SHADOWS CAST BY CONFUSED PEOPLE.

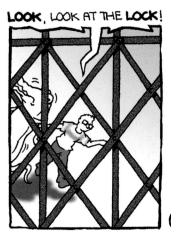

LOOK, LOOK AT THE **LOCK**!

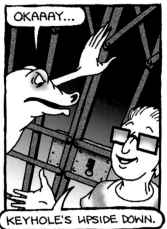

OKAAAY...

KEYHOLE'S UPSIDE DOWN.

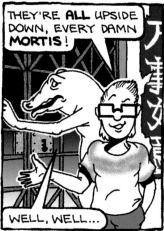

THEY'RE **ALL** UPSIDE DOWN, EVERY DAMN **MORTIS**!

WELL, WELL...

64

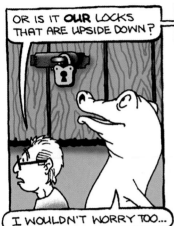

OR IS IT **OUR** LOCKS THAT ARE UPSIDE DOWN?

I WOULDN'T WORRY TOO...

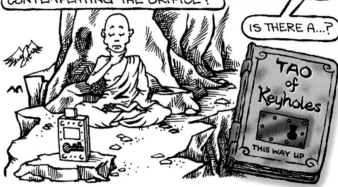

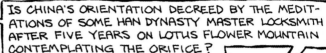

IS CHINA'S ORIENTATION DECREED BY THE MEDITATIONS OF SOME HAN DYNASTY MASTER LOCKSMITH AFTER FIVE YEARS ON LOTUS FLOWER MOUNTAIN CONTEMPLATING THE ORIFICE?

IS THERE A...?

TAO of Keyholes

THIS WAY UP

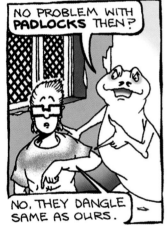

NO PROBLEM WITH **PADLOCKS** THEN?

NO, THEY DANGLE SAME AS OURS.

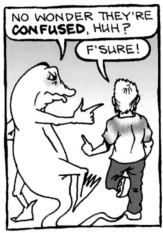

NO WONDER THEY'RE **CONFUSED**, HUH?

F'SURE!

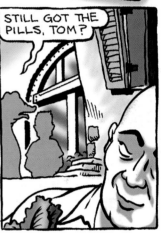

STILL GOT THE PILLS, TOM?

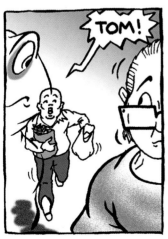

TOM!

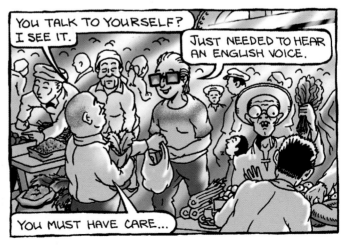

YOU TALK TO YOURSELF? I SEE IT.

JUST NEEDED TO HEAR AN ENGLISH VOICE.

YOU MUST HAVE CARE...

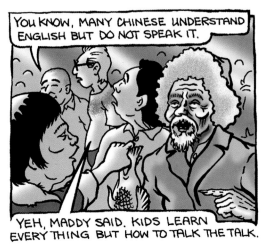

YOU KNOW, MANY CHINESE UNDERSTAND ENGLISH BUT DO NOT SPEAK IT.

YEH, MADDY SAID. KIDS LEARN EVERYTHING BUT HOW TO TALK THE TALK.

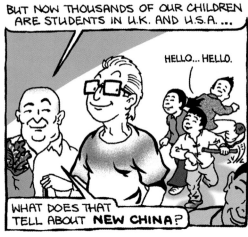

BUT NOW THOUSANDS OF OUR CHILDREN ARE STUDENTS IN U.K. AND U.S.A. ...

HELLO... HELLO.

WHAT DOES THAT TELL ABOUT **NEW CHINA**?

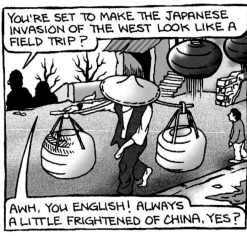

YOU'RE SET TO MAKE THE JAPANESE INVASION OF THE WEST LOOK LIKE A FIELD TRIP?

AWH, YOU ENGLISH! ALWAYS A LITTLE FRIGHTENED OF CHINA, YES?

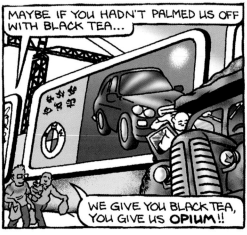

MAYBE IF YOU HADN'T PALMED US OFF WITH BLACK TEA...

WE GIVE YOU BLACK TEA, YOU GIVE US **OPIUM**!!

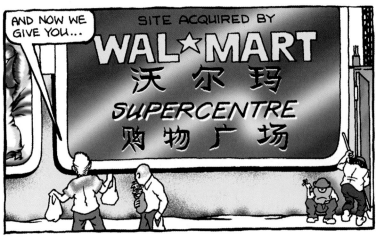

AND NOW WE GIVE YOU...

SITE ACQUIRED BY

WAL★MART

沃 尔 玛

SUPERCENTRE

购 物 广 场

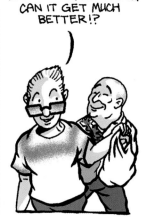

I ASK YOU, HONGXING, CAN IT GET MUCH BETTER!?

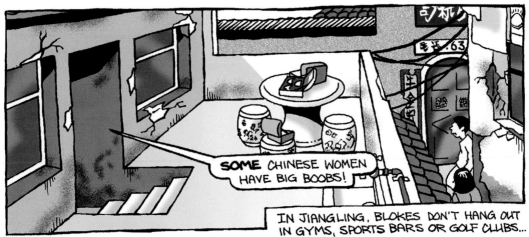

SOME CHINESE WOMEN HAVE BIG BOOBS!

IN JIANGLING, BLOKES DON'T HANG OUT IN GYMS, SPORTS BARS OR GOLF CLUBS...

THEY GO FOR A **MASSAGE**, THREE OR MORE TO A ROOM, WHICH WORRIED JUDY.

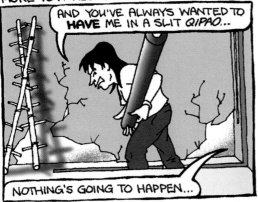

AND YOU'VE ALWAYS WANTED TO **HAVE** ME IN A SLIT *QIPAO*...

NOTHING'S GOING TO HAPPEN...

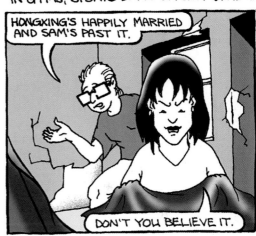

HONGXING'S HAPPILY MARRIED AND SAM'S PAST IT.

DON'T YOU BELIEVE IT.

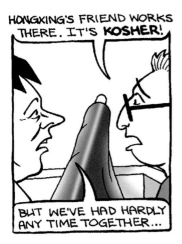

HONGXING'S FRIEND WORKS THERE. IT'S **KOSHER!**

BUT WE'VE HAD HARDLY ANY TIME TOGETHER...

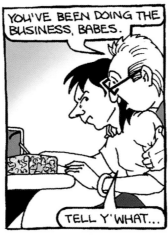

YOU'VE BEEN DOING THE BUSINESS, BABES.

TELL Y'WHAT...

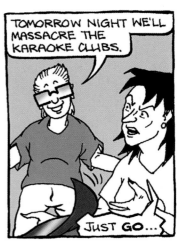

TOMORROW NIGHT WE'LL MASSACRE THE KARAOKE CLUBS.

JUST GO...

67

JIANGLING HAD SIX HOSPITALS, NO GPs AND ABOUT 30 FOOT MASSAGE PARLOURS, FREQUENTED AS A KIND OF PREVENTATIVE MEDICINE.

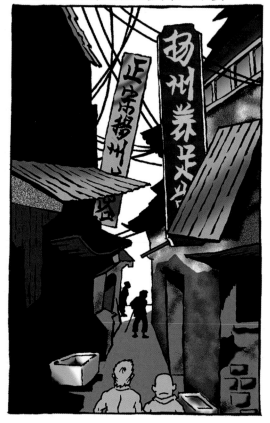

HONGXING CHOSE MASSEUSE NO. 42 AND GAVE ME HIS FRIEND, NO. 16.

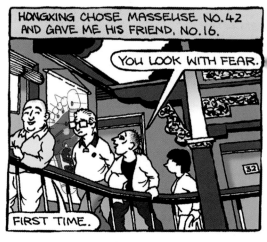

YOU LOOK WITH FEAR.

FIRST TIME.

WE WAITED BUT SAM DIDN'T SHOW.

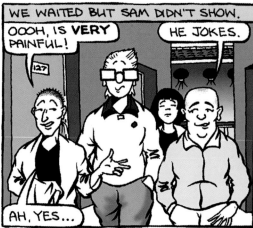

OOOH, IS **VERY** PAINFUL!

HE JOKES.

AH, YES...

HONGXING TELLS ME SHIT JOKE. GOOD ENGLISH JOKE, YES?

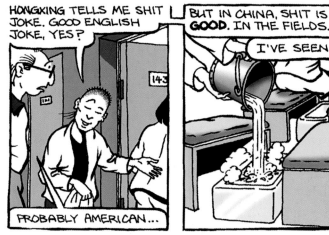

PROBABLY AMERICAN...

BUT IN CHINA, SHIT IS **GOOD**. IN THE FIELDS...

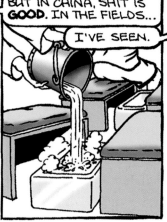

I'VE SEEN.

IT'S THE ONE THING ADMIRED BY EVERY TRAVELLER SINCE MARCO POLO, AND **STILL** WE HAVEN'T CAUGHT ON.

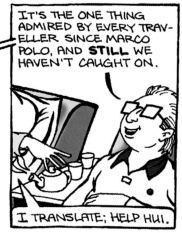

I TRANSLATE; HELP HUI.

HUI WAS ONE OF HONGXING'S OLD STUDENTS. A TALENTED CALIGRAPHER, HONGXING EXPECTED HIM TO BECOME A 'MOUNTAIN AND WATER' PAINTER.

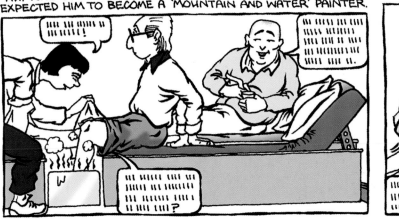

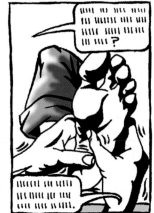

INSTEAD HE STUDIED WHAT THE WEST CALLS 'REFLEXOLOGY' UNDER A GRAND MASTER. "HE STILL BECOMES AN ARTIST," HONGXING PROUDLY TOLD ME.

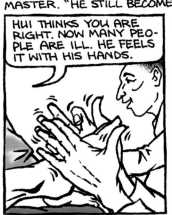

HUI THINKS YOU ARE RIGHT. NOW MANY PEOPLE ARE ILL. HE FEELS IT WITH HIS HANDS.

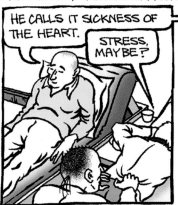

HE CALLS IT SICKNESS OF THE HEART.

STRESS, MAYBE?

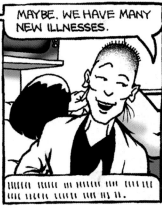

MAYBE. WE HAVE MANY NEW ILLNESSES.

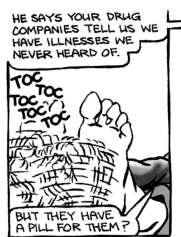

HE SAYS YOUR DRUG COMPANIES TELL US WE HAVE ILLNESSES WE NEVER HEARD OF.

TOC TOC TOC TOC TOC

BUT THEY HAVE A PILL FOR THEM?

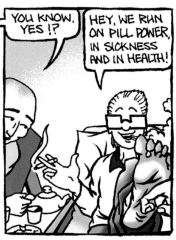

YOU KNOW, YES !?

HEY, WE RUN ON PILL POWER, IN SICKNESS AND IN HEALTH!

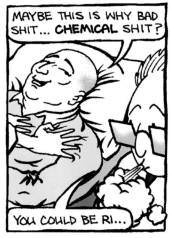

MAYBE THIS IS WHY BAD SHIT... **CHEMICAL** SHIT?

YOU COULD BE RI...

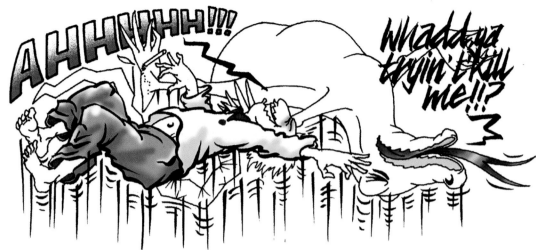

AHHHHHH!!!

Whaddaya tryin' t' kill me!!?

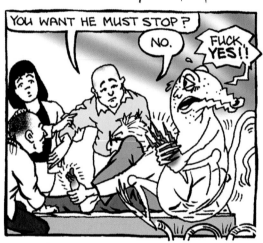

YOU WANT HE MUST STOP?

NO.

FUCK YES!!

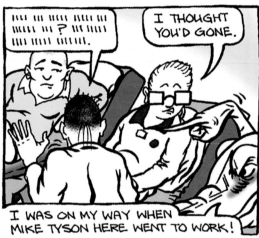

IIII III IIIII IIIII III IIIIII III ? III IIIII IIIII IIIII IIIIII.

I THOUGHT YOU'D GONE.

I WAS ON MY WAY WHEN MIKE TYSON HERE WENT TO WORK!

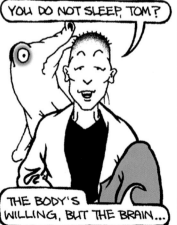

YOU DO NOT SLEEP, TOM?

THE BODY'S WILLING, BUT THE BRAIN...

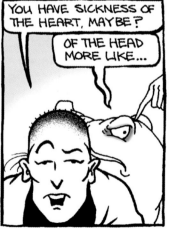

YOU HAVE SICKNESS OF THE HEART, MAYBE?

OF THE HEAD MORE LIKE...

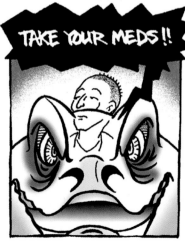

TAKE YOUR MEDS!!

WHERE THE WEST SEP-
ARATES MIND FROM BODY
AND LOST SIGHT OF THE
SOUL CENTURIES AGO, THE
EAST CONSIDERS THE
PATIENT A COMPLETE
BEING, PART OF THE UNI-
VERSE.

WHILE WE DISH OUT
PILLS AND POTIONS, THEY
TWEEK THE BODY'S *QI*
(VITAL ENERGY), EQUAL-
ISING *YIN* AND *YANG*,
INSIDE AND OUT, BALANC-
ING THE FIVE ELEMENTS.

OUR HEAD CASES ARE
HOSPITISED, ISOLATED IN
THE COMMUNITY, CONSIGN-
ED TO A CHEMICAL STRAIT-
JACKET. THEIRS ARE CARED FOR IN BIG
FAMILIES AND CLOSE COMMUNITIES, TREAT-
ED WITH TRADITIONAL MEDICINES AND
THERAPIES LIKE ACUPUNCTURE, MOXIBUSTION
AND MASSAGE.

OR THEY WERE...

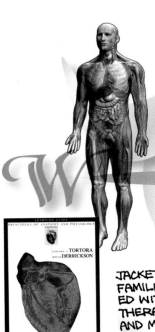

PRINCIPLES OF ANATOMY
AND PHYSIOLOGY (1983)

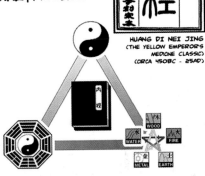

HUANG DI NEI JING
(THE YELLOW EMPEROR'S
MEDICINE CLASSIC)
(CIRCA 450BC - 25AD)

UNTIL VERY RECENTLY, THERE WAS NO
CHINESE WORD FOR DEPRESSION. *YU*
(GLOOMY), *YI* (REPRESSED) AND *ZHENG*
(DISORDER) WERE ALL EMPLOYED UNDER
THE UMBRELLA OF *SHENJING SHUAIRUO*
(NEUROLOGICAL WEAKNESS), A DIAGNOSIS
SO BROAD IT CARRIED NO STIGMA.

ANYTHING MORE SPECIFIC WAS
DESCRIBED AS A SYMPTOM OF A PART-
ICULAR ORGAN, LIKE THE LIVER, HEART
OR SPLEEN. NOT THAT IT WASN'T FUN-
CTIONING, BUT IT WAS A RELUCTANT
PARTICIPANT CAPABLE OF INFECTING
THE WHOLE SYSTEM WITH ITS NEGATIVE
VIBES.

A SICKNESS OF THE HEART
DECIDED HUI TO BECOME A
HEALER - THE SICKNESS OF
HIS FATHER.

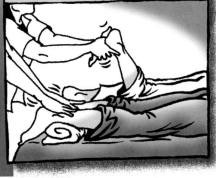

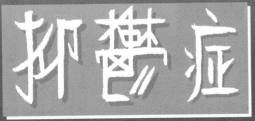

71

AS A NAIVE RED GUARD, HUI'S DAD DENOUNCED HIS ELDEST BROTHER AT A MASS SHAMING IN WHAT WAS THEN RED SQUARE.

THE BROTHER WAS DESPATCHED TO A LABOUR CAMP IN GANSU PROVINCE, NEVER TO BE HEARD OF AGAIN.

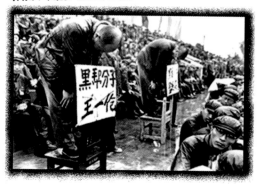

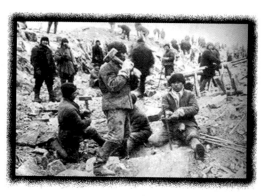

HUI'S DAD WAS CONSUMED WITH GUILT AND PLAGUED WITH DEPRESSION FOR THE REST OF HIS LIFE.

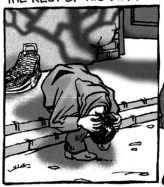

EXCEPT THAT THE PEOPLE OF THE PEOPLE'S REPUBLIC DIDN'T SUFFER FROM SICKNESSES OF THE HEART, 'COS CHAIRMAN MAO SAID SO.

DEPRESSION IS A BOURGEOIS SELF-INDULGENCE BORN OF **INCORRECT** POLITICAL THINKING.

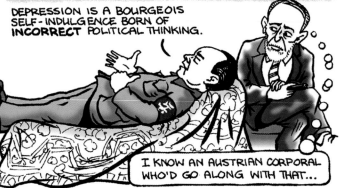

I KNOW AN AUSTRIAN CORPORAL WHO'D GO ALONG WITH THAT...

HUNDREDS OF **MILLIONS** OF CHINESE WERE TRAUMATISED BY THE REVOLUTION. ASIDE FROM THE HEADLINE HORRORS, FAMILY AND COMMUNITY BONDS WERE RIPPED APART, DEMOLISHING THE TRADITIONAL SANCTUARY FOR THE WEAK OF QI.

AND IF SICKNESSES OF THE HEART WERE ONCE FREE OF THE STIGMA MENTAL ILLNESS HAS IN THE WEST, MAO'S DOGMA ENSURED CHINA'S PSYCHOS NO LONGER MISSED OUT. THEY STILL SUFFER IN SILENCE.

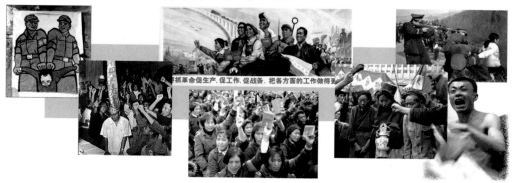

When Deng Xiaoping finally acknowledged a few more comrades than Hui's dad were down with the bourgeois blues, China began the painfully slow process of building a modern mental health service along western lines (some say more to appease the human rights lobby than the demand).

Hui took the short cut, training to do what he had secretly been doing for his father for years.

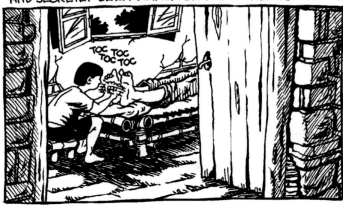

TOC TOC
TOC TOC

Twenty years on, there are more renminbi billionaires than state psychotherapists in China. Traditional therapies are back in favour for prevention as much as cure, but families and communites are increasingly fractured, now by the economic revolution.

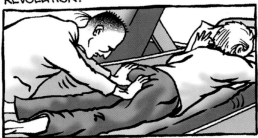

Depression is a factor in 1-in-4 homicides. Men mostly murder wives or lovers, women almost exclusively kill their 'little emperors', the spoilt brats born of the **one-child policy**. China is now **2nd** in the world suicide league and **top** of the women's table.

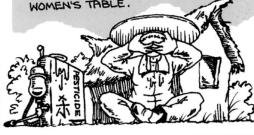

PESTICIDE

And now we have **Morita therapy**.

Which we do not talk of.

We don't?

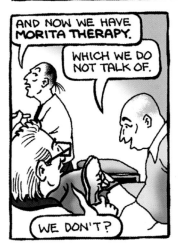

It is **Japanese**.

43

?

Don't go there...

What the Germans are to the Brits, the Japs are to the Chinese, with a vengeance.

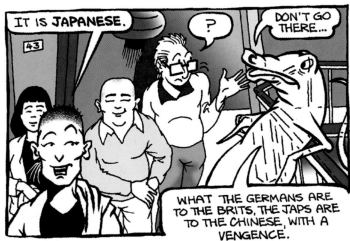

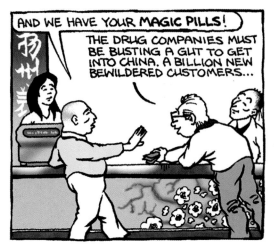

AND WE HAVE YOUR **MAGIC PILLS**!

THE DRUG COMPANIES MUST BE BUSTING A GUT TO GET INTO CHINA. A BILLION NEW BEWILDERED CUSTOMERS...

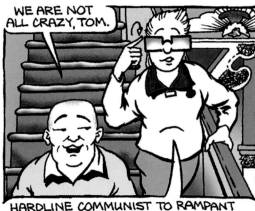

WE ARE NOT ALL CRAZY, TOM.

HARDLINE COMMUNIST TO RAMPANT CAPITALIST IN LESS THAN A LIFETIME? IT'D DO MY HEAD IN...

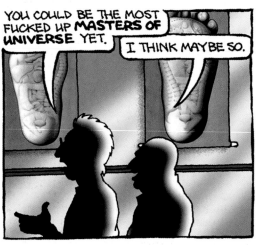

YOU COULD BE THE MOST FUCKED UP **MASTERS OF UNIVERSE** YET.

I THINK MAYBE SO.

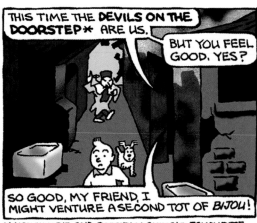

THIS TIME THE **DEVILS ON THE DOORSTEP**✳ ARE US.

BUT YOU FEEL GOOD, YES?

SO GOOD, MY FRIEND, I MIGHT VENTURE A SECOND TOT OF *BIJOU*!

✳ HONGXING'S AND POSSIBLY CHINA'S FAVOURITE FILM, ABOUT STICKING IT TO THE JAPS IN WWII.

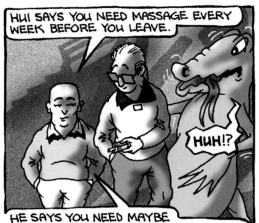

HUI SAYS YOU NEED MASSAGE EVERY WEEK BEFORE YOU LEAVE.

HUH!?

HE SAYS YOU NEED MAYBE SIX MONTHS, BUT HE CAN HELP YOU...

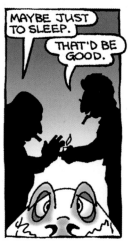

MAYBE JUST TO SLEEP.

THAT'D BE GOOD.

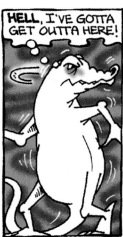

HELL, I'VE GOTTA GET OUTTA HERE!

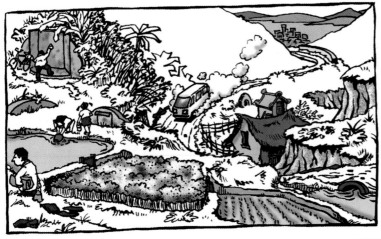

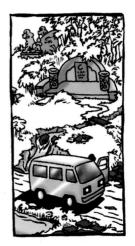

It was **QING MING JIE**, ANCESTOR'S DAY, WHEN THE GRAVES ARE CLEANED. WE WERE JOINED BY NUYING'S SON, FENG.

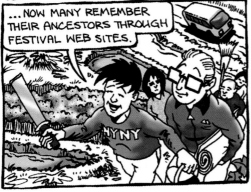

...NOW MANY REMEMBER THEIR ANCESTORS THROUGH FESTIVAL WEB SITES.

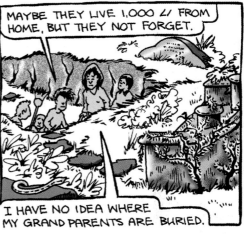

MAYBE THEY LIVE 1,000 *LI* FROM HOME, BUT THEY NOT FORGET.

I HAVE NO IDEA WHERE MY GRANDPARENTS ARE BURIED.

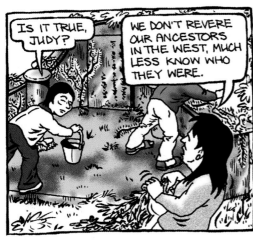

IS IT TRUE, JUDY?

WE DON'T REVERE OUR ANCESTORS IN THE WEST, MUCH LESS KNOW WHO THEY WERE.

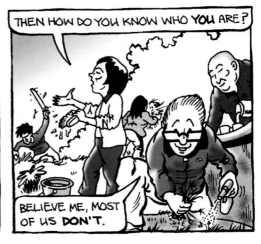

THEN HOW DO YOU KNOW WHO **YOU** ARE?

BELIEVE ME, MOST OF US **DON'T**.

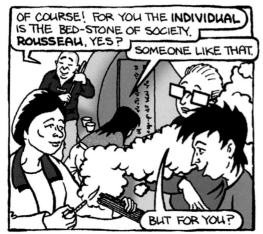

OF COURSE! FOR YOU THE **INDIVIDUAL** IS THE BED-STONE OF SOCIETY. **ROUSSEAU**, YES?

SOMEONE LIKE THAT.

BUT FOR YOU?

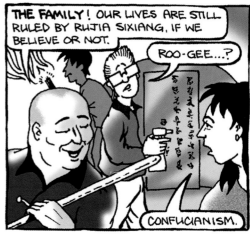

THE FAMILY! OUR LIVES ARE STILL RULED BY RUJIA SIXIANG, IF WE BELIEVE OR NOT.

ROO-GEE...?

CONFUCIANISM.

ORIGINALLY A CODE OF CONDUCT, CONFUCIANISM IS MORE A PHILOSOPHY THAN RELIGION. THE DEFINING HEADSET FOR 2,500 YEARS, IT PREACHES THE CONCEPT OF 'SAVING FACE' THAT HAS MADE THE CHINESE EMOTIONALLY RESTRAINED, AND THAT RESPECT FLOWS UPWARDS, YOUNG TO OLD, SUBJECT TO RULER. DEFINING PATTERNS OF BEHAVIOUR, IT PLAYED INTO THE HANDS OF THE DYNASTIES, PLACING THE FAMILY AND STATE AT THE CENTRE OF PRE-COMMUNIST SOCIETY. BUT AS HONGXING PUT IT...

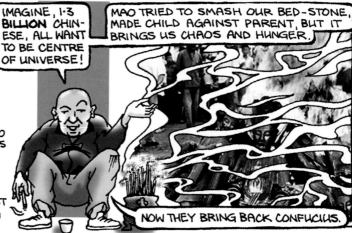

IMAGINE, 1.3 **BILLION** CHINESE, ALL WANT TO BE CENTRE OF UNIVERSE!

MAO TRIED TO SMASH OUR BED-STONE, MADE CHILD AGAINST PARENT, BUT IT BRINGS US CHAOS AND HUNGER.

NOW THEY BRING BACK CONFUCIUS.

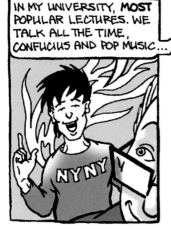

IN MY UNIVERSITY, **MOST** POPULAR LECTURES. WE TALK ALL THE TIME, CONFUCIUS AND POP MUSIC...

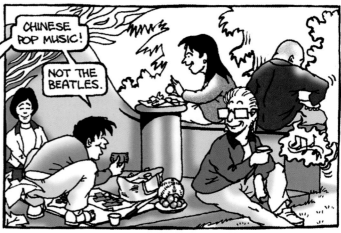

CHINESE POP MUSIC!

NOT THE BEATLES.

NYNY

76

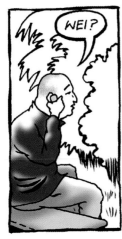

WEI?

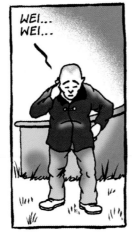

WEI... WEI...

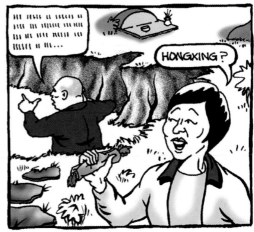

HONGXING?

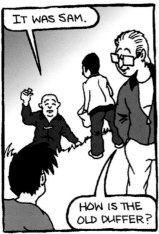

IT WAS SAM.

HOW IS THE OLD DUFFER?

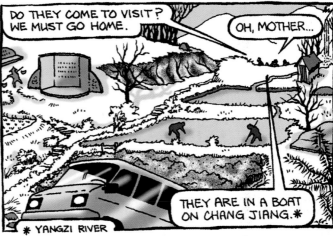

DO THEY COME TO VISIT? WE MUST GO HOME.

OH, MOTHER...

THEY ARE IN A BOAT ON CHANG JIANG.*

* YANGZI RIVER

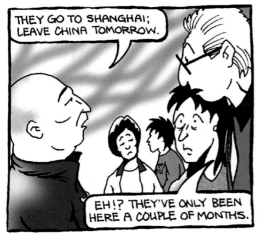

THEY GO TO SHANGHAI; LEAVE CHINA TOMORROW.

EH!? THEY'VE ONLY BEEN HERE A COUPLE OF MONTHS.

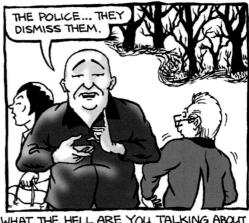

THE POLICE... THEY DISMISS THEM.

WHAT THE HELL ARE YOU TALKING ABOUT?

SAM AND MADDY HAD FALLEN FOUL OF THE **GOLD SHIELD PROJECT**, THE INTELLIGENCE MACHINE THAT KEEPS THE PEOPLE'S REPUBLIC IN CHECK.

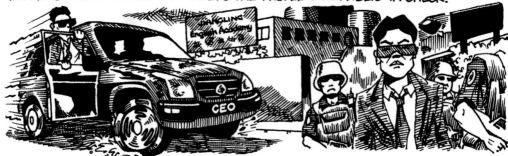

THE STORY GOES THAT THEY WERE WORKING UNDER TOURIST VISAS. THE DIRECTOR OF THE ACADEMY WAS SUPPOSED TO BE PULLING STRINGS TO GET THEM WORK VISAS BUT THE SPECIAL POLICE UNIT CAUGHT WIND.

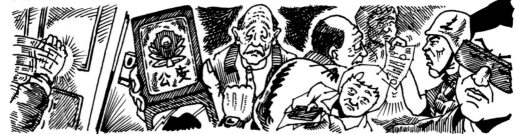

ON THE NIGHT OF THE FOOT MASSAGE, THEY PAID A VISIT. BY THREE THE NEXT MORNING, SAM AND MADDY WERE STEAMING DOWNSTREAM.

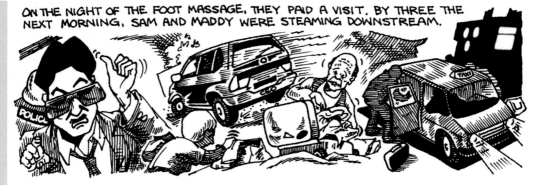

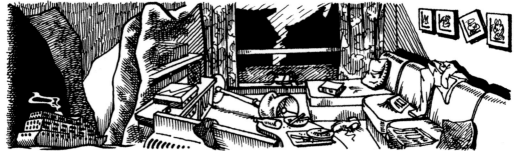

THEY LEFT EVERYTHING, INCLUDING MOST OF THEIR CLOTHES.

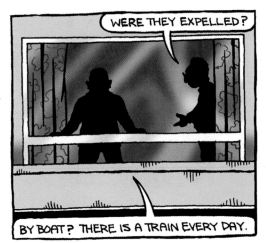

WERE THEY EXPELLED?

BY BOAT? THERE IS A TRAIN EVERY DAY.

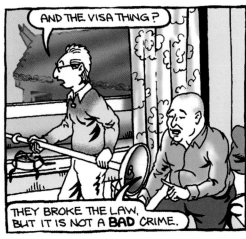

AND THE VISA THING?

THEY BROKE THE LAW, BUT IT IS NOT A **BAD** CRIME.

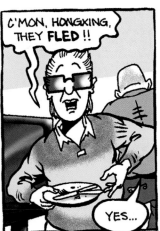

C'MON, HONGXING, THEY **FLED**!!

YES...

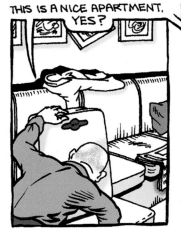

THIS IS A NICE APARTMENT, YES?

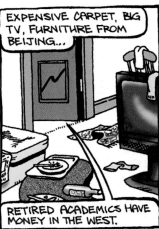

EXPENSIVE CARPET, BIG TV, FURNITURE FROM BEIJING...

RETIRED ACADEMICS HAVE MONEY IN THE WEST.

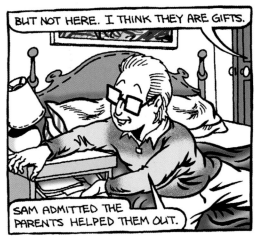

BUT NOT HERE. I THINK THEY ARE GIFTS.

SAM ADMITTED THE PARENTS HELPED THEM OUT.

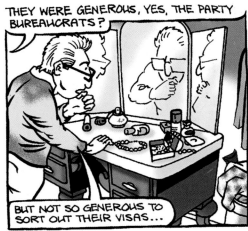

THEY WERE GENEROUS, YES, THE PARTY BUREAUCRATS?

BUT NOT SO GENEROUS TO SORT OUT THEIR VISAS...

79

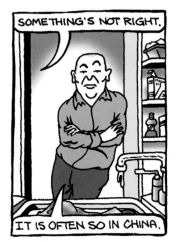

SOMETHING'S NOT RIGHT.

IT IS OFTEN SO IN CHINA.

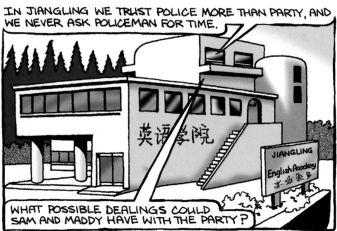

IN JIANGLING WE TRUST POLICE MORE THAN PARTY, AND WE NEVER ASK POLICEMAN FOR TIME.

英语学院

JIANGLING English Academy

WHAT POSSIBLE DEALINGS COULD SAM AND MADDY HAVE WITH THE PARTY?

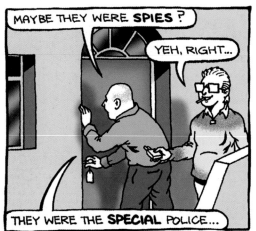

MAYBE THEY WERE **SPIES**?

YEH, RIGHT...

THEY WERE THE **SPECIAL** POLICE...

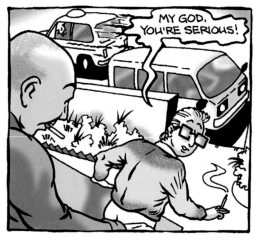

MY GOD, YOU'RE SERIOUS!

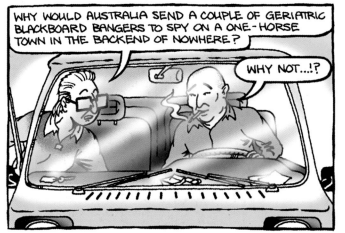

WHY WOULD AUSTRALIA SEND A COUPLE OF GERIATRIC BLACKBOARD BANGERS TO SPY ON A ONE-HORSE TOWN IN THE BACKEND OF NOWHERE?

WHY NOT...!?

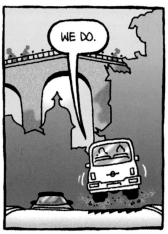

WE DO.

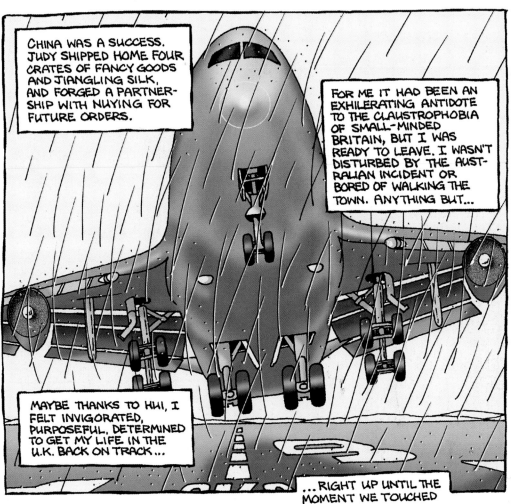

CHINA WAS A SUCCESS. JUDY SHIPPED HOME FOUR CRATES OF FANCY GOODS AND JIANGLING SILK, AND FORGED A PARTNERSHIP WITH NUYING FOR FUTURE ORDERS.

FOR ME IT HAD BEEN AN EXHILERATING ANTIDOTE TO THE CLAUSTROPHOBIA OF SMALL-MINDED BRITAIN, BUT I WAS READY TO LEAVE. I WASN'T DISTURBED BY THE AUSTRALIAN INCIDENT OR BORED OF WALKING THE TOWN. ANYTHING BUT...

MAYBE THANKS TO HUI, I FELT INVIGORATED, PURPOSEFUL, DETERMINED TO GET MY LIFE IN THE U.K. BACK ON TRACK...

...RIGHT UP UNTIL THE MOMENT WE TOUCHED DOWN.

Graveyard Shift

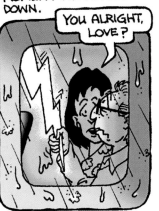

YOU ALRIGHT, LOVE?

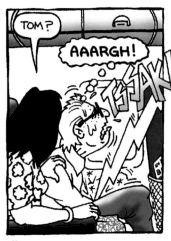

TOM?

AAARGH!

TSSAK!

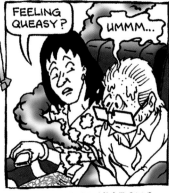

FEELING QUEASY?

UMMM...

ACCORDING TO MY BALLS, I WAS ON THE VERGE OF A **CATACLYSMIC** BREAKDOWN.

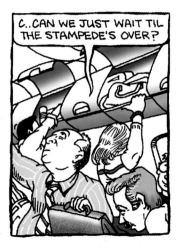

C..CAN WE JUST WAIT TIL THE STAMPEDE'S OVER?

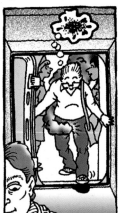

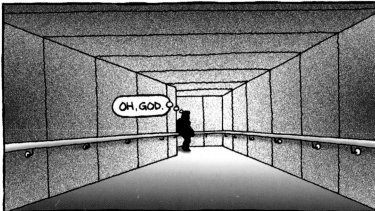

OH, GOD.

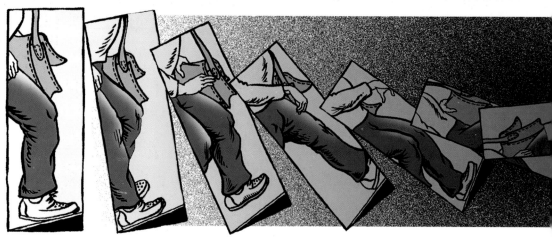

EVERY STEP UP THE BOARDING BRIDGE TO THE TERMINAL DROPPED ME DEEPER DOWN THE BLACK HOLE OF DESPONDENCY.

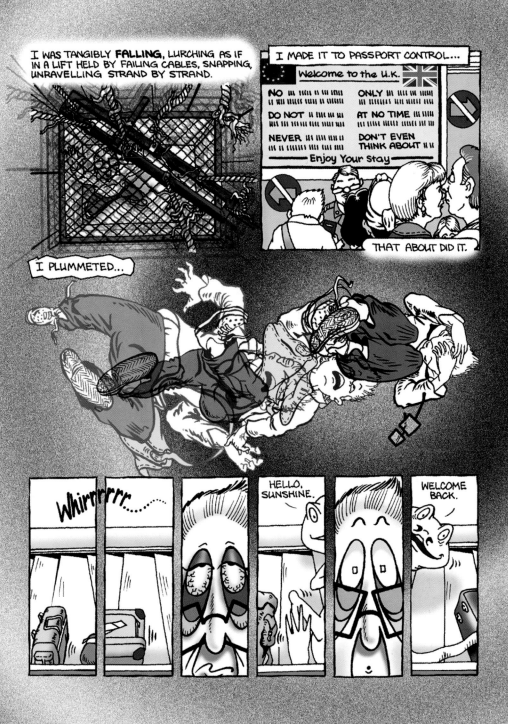

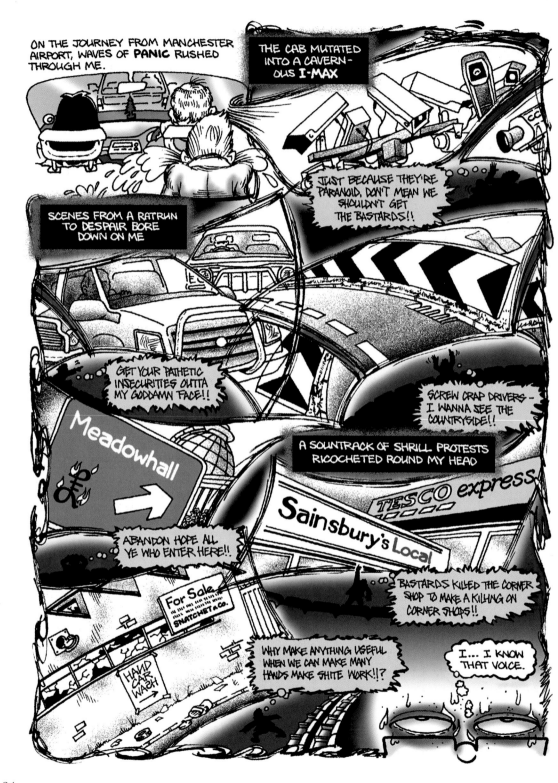

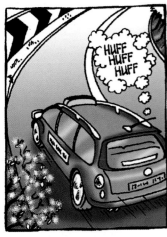

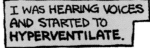
I WAS HEARING VOICES AND STARTED TO **HYPERVENTILATE.**

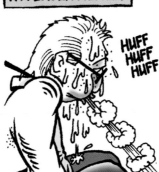

MY HANDS BEGAN ROTATING LIKE FEET CLIPPED IN PEDALS.

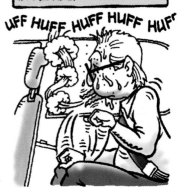

I WAS TOILING OVER HILL AND DALE, GRINDING UP ESCARPMENTS, FIGHTING HEAD WINDS ON THE DOWN. **OF COURSE** I WAS GASPING FOR AIR, BUT I HAD DONE THIS A MILLION TIMES.

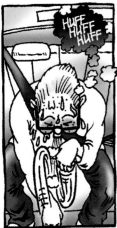

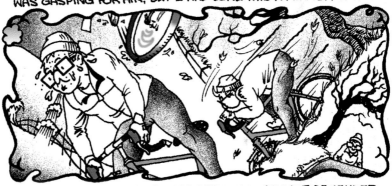

I KNEW HOW TO STABILISE MY BREATHING. COULD I REMEMBER...

WHEN WE ARRIVED HOME...

I'VE GOTTA GO TO BED, JUDY.

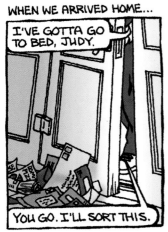

YOU GO. I'LL SORT THIS.

TEN-TO-ONE, IF THE CATERING DOESN'T GET YOU THE JET LAG WILL.

I'LL MAKE US A BREW...

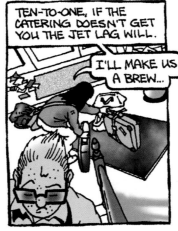

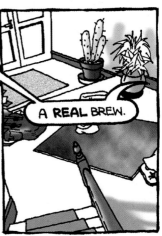

A **REAL** BREW.

85

ONE THING I LEARNED FROM MY EARLIER ENCOUNTER WITH THE BIG D., IF YOU ARE FEELING DEPRESSED, CHANCES ARE YOU AIN'T **DEPRESSED**. THE REAL McCOY DEFIES EXPRESSION. IT HURLS YOUR EVERY EMOTION INTO AN INDUSTRIAL MIXER THAT REDUCES ALL FEELING TO AN INDESCRIBABLE **GLOB**. THE BEST YOU CAN SAY IS THAT BEING DEPRESSED IS **SHIT**, UNLESS YOU LIKE BEING ENTOMBED IN WET, SHRINKING CONCRETE.

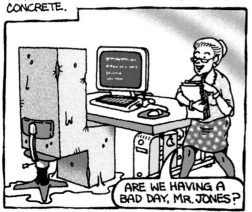

ARE WE HAVING A BAD DAY, MR. JONES?

EXCEPT FOR SURFING WAVE UPON WAVE OF NEGATIVE THOUGHTS, I WAS MENTALLY PARALYSED.

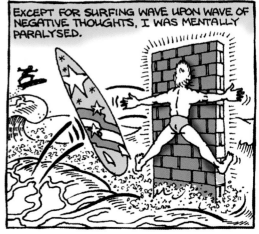

PHYSICALLY, THERE WERE FOETAL DAYS, WEEKS EVEN, WHEN STAMPEDING WILDER- BEAST COULDN'T HAVE MADE ME UNCOIL MY LIMBS.

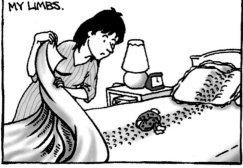

IF I FELT ANYTHING, IT WAS **FEAR** LIKE I HAVE NEVER KNOWN. A TERROR THAT TRANS- PORTED ME TO PLACES WAY OFF MY MAP.

FORGIVE ME FATHER, I MUST HAVE SINNED.

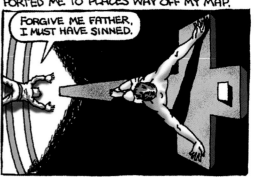

IT **WAS** LIKE A PART OF ME HAD DIED, A PART I NEVER KNEW.

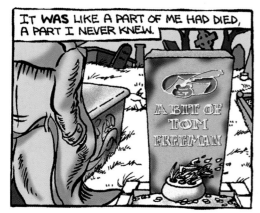

A BIT OF TOM FREEMAN

I WAS CONSUMED BY AN OVER-POWERING SENSE OF **LOSS** AND **SADNESS**.

FAREWELL, MY FRIEND, I WISH WE'D MET.

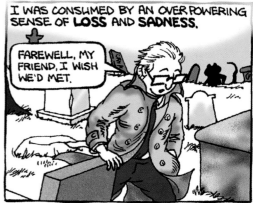

86

BEWILDERING, HUH?

THOROUGHLY.

THE PINS THAT HOLD YOUR LIFE TOGETHER HAVE BEEN DISLODGED...

SPAT OUT BY A **FEROCIOUS** BUILD UP OF **PRESSURE.**

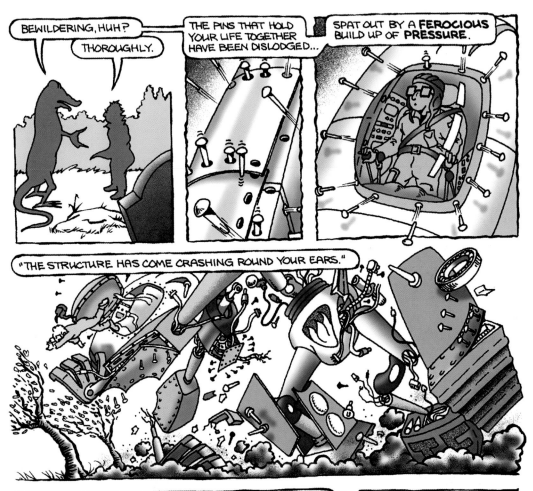

"THE STRUCTURE HAS COME CRASHING ROUND YOUR EARS."

"YOU HAVE SURVIVED THE FALL BUT ABOUT YOU LIES THE DEBRIS OF A LIFE ONCE ORDERED AND ARRANGED."

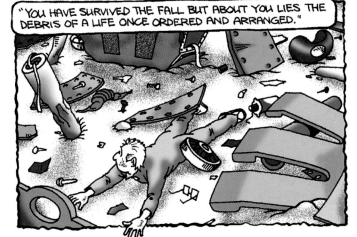

SO I'M **DERANGED?**

LET'S JUST SAY SOMEWHAT **PIXILATED.**

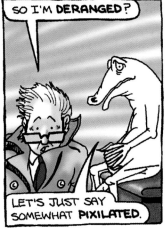

87

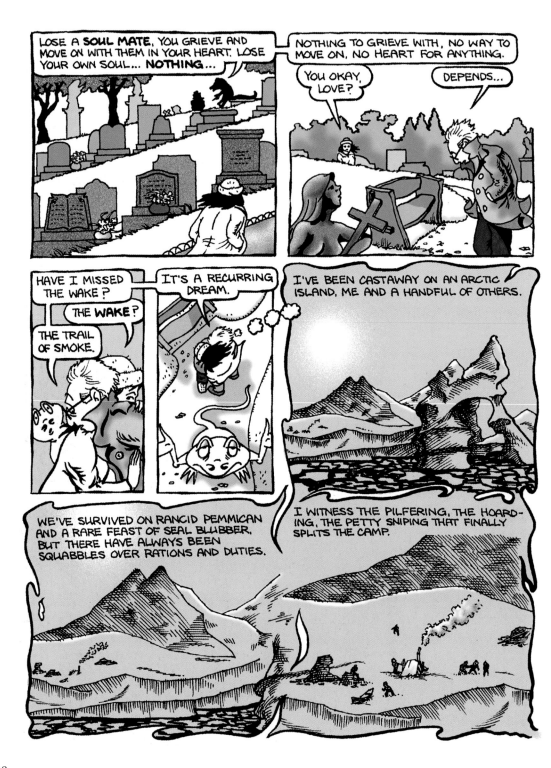

LOSE A **SOUL MATE**, YOU GRIEVE AND MOVE ON WITH THEM IN YOUR HEART. LOSE YOUR OWN SOUL... **NOTHING**...

NOTHING TO GRIEVE WITH, NO WAY TO MOVE ON, NO HEART FOR ANYTHING.

YOU OKAY, LOVE?

DEPENDS...

HAVE I MISSED THE WAKE?

THE **WAKE**?

THE TRAIL OF SMOKE.

IT'S A RECURRING DREAM.

I'VE BEEN CASTAWAY ON AN ARCTIC ISLAND, ME AND A HANDFUL OF OTHERS.

WE'VE SURVIVED ON RANCID PEMMICAN AND A RARE FEAST OF SEAL BLUBBER, BUT THERE HAVE ALWAYS BEEN SQUABBLES OVER RATIONS AND DUTIES.

I WITNESS THE PILFERING, THE HOARDING, THE PETTY SNIPING THAT FINALLY SPLITS THE CAMP.

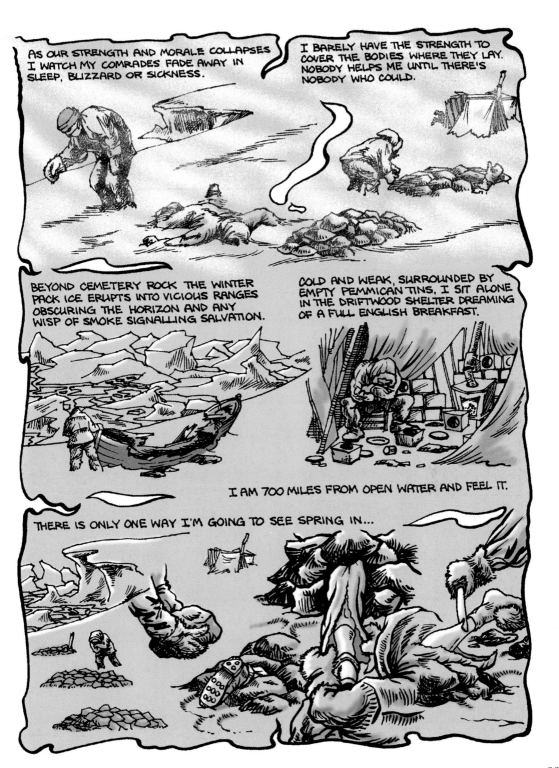

AS OUR STRENGTH AND MORALE COLLAPSES I WATCH MY COMRADES FADE AWAY IN SLEEP, BLIZZARD OR SICKNESS.

I BARELY HAVE THE STRENGTH TO COVER THE BODIES WHERE THEY LAY. NOBODY HELPS ME UNTIL THERE'S NOBODY WHO COULD.

BEYOND CEMETERY ROCK THE WINTER PACK ICE ERUPTS INTO VICIOUS RANGES OBSCURING THE HORIZON AND ANY WISP OF SMOKE SIGNALLING SALVATION.

COLD AND WEAK, SURROUNDED BY EMPTY PEMMICAN TINS, I SIT ALONE IN THE DRIFTWOOD SHELTER DREAMING OF A FULL ENGLISH BREAKFAST.

I AM 700 MILES FROM OPEN WATER AND FEEL IT.

THERE IS ONLY ONE WAY I'M GOING TO SEE SPRING IN...

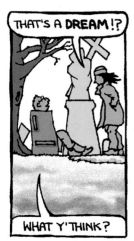

THAT'S A **DREAM**!?

WHAT Y'THINK?

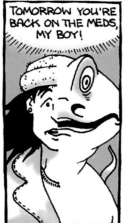

TOMORROW YOU'RE BACK ON THE MEDS, MY BOY!

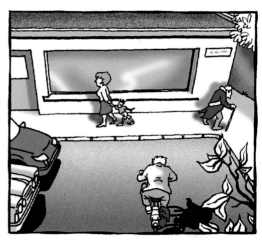

IT WAS MATTERHORN'S DAY OFF.

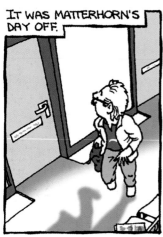

I WAS PASSED ON TO A **THIRD** DOCTOR – YOUNG, EAGER AND A BAG OF NERVES.

COME IN, ER... TOM.

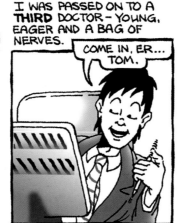

HE CLICKED AND FLICKED INCESSANTLY, SCROLLING THROUGH MY RECORDS LIKE AN ASPERGERS WITH AN XBOX.

REMARKABLE, QUITE REMARKABLE!

BEFORE YOU JOINED US YOUR ONLY CONTACT WITH THE HEALTH SERVICE WAS FOR BREAKS, FRACTURES, CARTILAGES AND **MALARIA.**

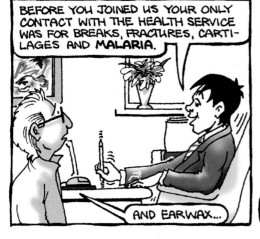

AND EARWAX...

IS THERE SOMETHING ABOUT YOUR PROFESSION I SHOULD KNOW, TOM?

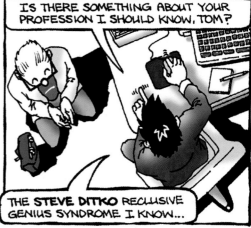

THE **STEVE DITKO** RECLUSIVE GENIUS SYNDROME. I KNOW...

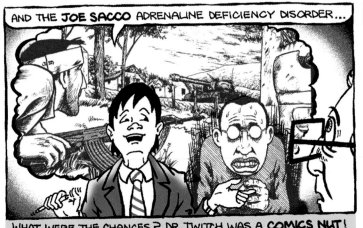

AND THE **JOE SACCO** ADRENALINE DEFICIENCY DISORDER...

WHAT WERE THE CHANCES? DR. TWITCH WAS A **COMICS NUT!**

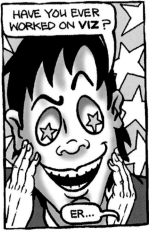

HAVE YOU EVER WORKED ON **VIZ**?

ER...

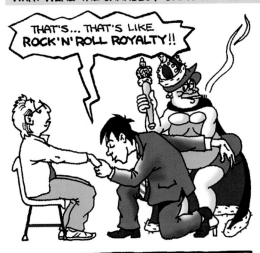

THAT'S... THAT'S LIKE **ROCK'N'ROLL ROYALTY!!**

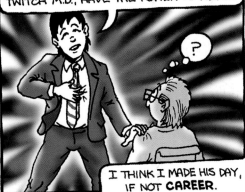

BEFORE ME SLUMPS THE SHELL OF A BROKEN CARTOONIST WHO **I**, NIGEL TWITCH M.D., HAVE THE POWER TO **HEAL**.

?

I THINK I MADE HIS DAY, IF NOT **CAREER**.

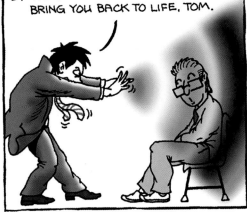

BY THE HOSTS OF **HOGGOTH**, I WILL BRING YOU BACK TO LIFE, TOM.

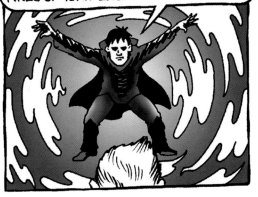

I WILL PUT **LEAD** IN YOU PENCIL AND **INK** IN YOUR VEINS, REKINDLE THE FIRES OF YOUR **EXQUISITE CREATIVITY**...

91

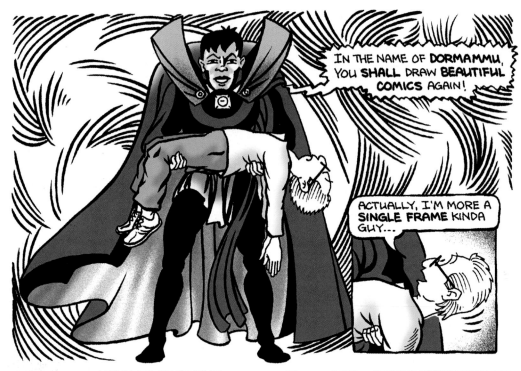

IN THE NAME OF **DORMAMMU**, YOU **SHALL** DRAW **BEAUTIFUL COMICS** AGAIN!

ACTUALLY, I'M MORE A **SINGLE FRAME** KINDA GUY...

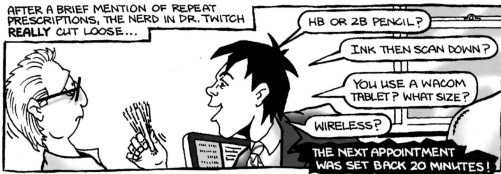

AFTER A BRIEF MENTION OF REPEAT PRESCRIPTIONS, THE NERD IN DR. TWITCH **REALLY** CUT LOOSE...

HB OR 2B PENCIL?

INK THEN SCAN DOWN?

YOU USE A WACOM TABLET? WHAT SIZE?

WIRELESS?

THE NEXT APPOINTMENT WAS SET BACK 20 MINUTES!

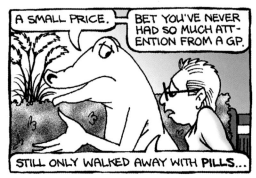

A SMALL PRICE.

BET YOU'VE NEVER HAD SO MUCH ATT-ENTION FROM A G.P.

STILL ONLY WALKED AWAY WITH **PILLS**...

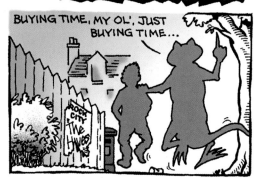

BUYING TIME, MY OL', JUST BUYING TIME....

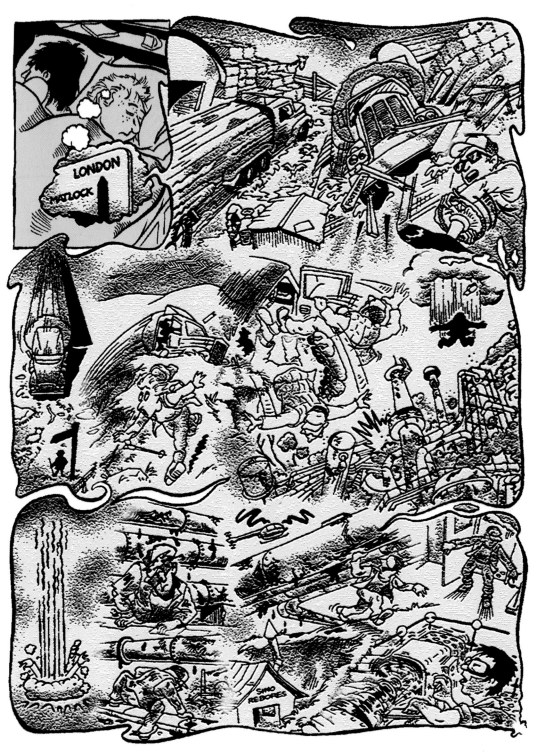

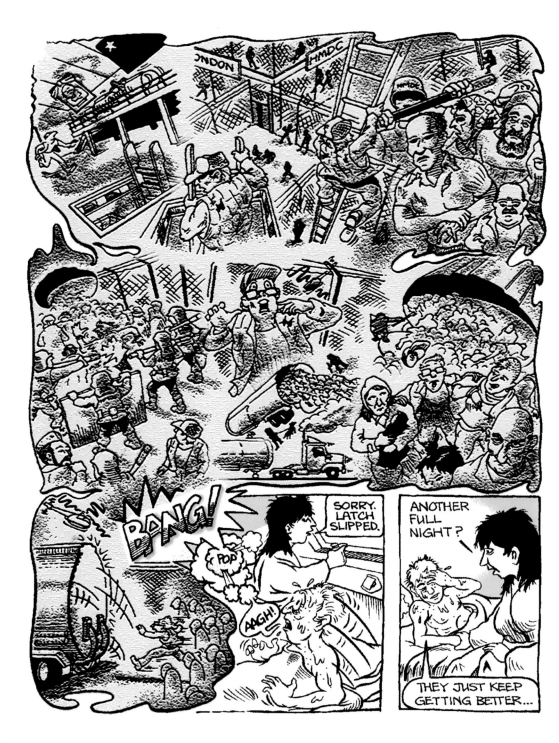

IT SEEMS LIKE I HAVE ALWAYS HAD DISTURBED NIGHTS, CERTAINLY SINCE MY THREE-LEGGED DOG DIED IN HER SLEEP FOR NO APPARENT REASON.

PEG WAS A PLUCKY LITTLE LASS. SHE LOST HER LEG IN AN ARGUMENT WITH A THUG OF A ROTTWEILLER WHOSE OWNER SHOULD HAVE BEEN ON THE RECEIVING END OF THE LETHAL INJECTION.

DISABLED MOST OF HER LIFE, PEG CLIMBED MOUNTAINS WITH ME, OR WHAT A TEN YEAR OLD WOULD CALL MOUNTAINS.

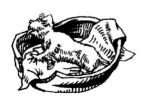 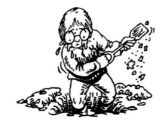 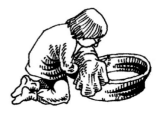

SHE WAS THE FIRST FLESH AND BLOOD I TRULY LOVED. I WAS DECIMATED WHEN DEATH STOLE HER AWAY WITHOUT WARNING.

FOR YEARS I FEARED THE SAME FATE AND FOUGHT SLEEP, THOUGH THE LONGEST I WENT WITHOUT WAS FOUR DAYS (IN MY TEENS AND SWIMMING IN STIMULANTS).

EVEN NOW, WHEN MY HEAD HITS THE PILLOW, I RATTLE THROUGH UNFINISHED BUSINESS, BUILDING AN APPEAL TO MORT'S MERCIFUL SIDE.

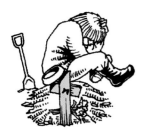 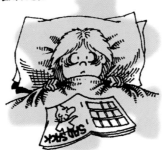 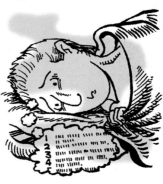

IF I GET UP FOR A PEE, I RUN THROUGH THE LIST OF MITIGATIONS AGAIN BEFORE ALLOWING SLEEP TO RETURN.

THESE ARE NOT THE CIRCUMSTANCES CONDUSIVE TO TECHNICOLOUR DREAMS OF BUTTERFLIES AND SWAYING CORN.

THE MEDS WERE SUPPOSED TO SMOTHER MY ANXIETIES, KNOCK ME OUT, DO **SOMETHING**.

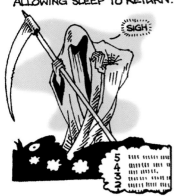 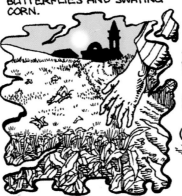 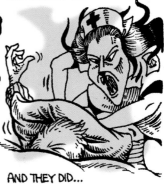

AND THEY DID...

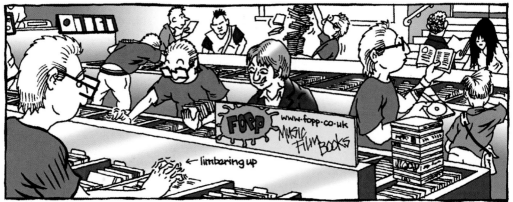

AFTER A LIFE-TIME OF BEING A RELUCTANT SHOPPER, I SUDDENLY BECAME A **COMPULSIVE CONSUMER**, ALBEIT SELECTIVE-COMPULSIVE – MUSIC, FILMS, BOOKS, COMICS.

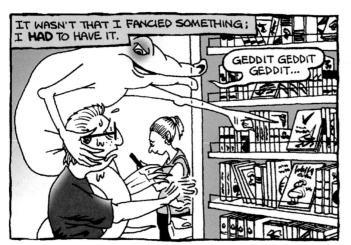

IT WASN'T THAT I FANCIED SOMETHING; I **HAD** TO HAVE IT.

GEDDIT GEDDIT GEDDIT...

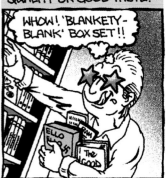

AND MY CRAVINGS WERE NOT ENCUMBERED BY ANYTHING SO SNIFFY AS QUALITY OR GOOD TASTE.

WHOW! 'BLANKETY-BLANK' BOX SET!!

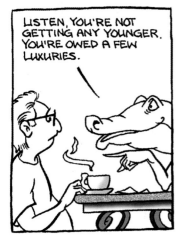

LISTEN, YOU'RE NOT GETTING ANY YOUNGER. YOU'RE OWED A FEW LUXURIES.

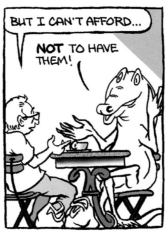

BUT I CAN'T AFFORD...

NOT TO HAVE THEM!

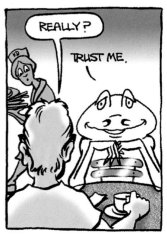

REALLY?

TRUST ME.

96

I COULDN'T DO A SUPERMARKET RUN WITHOUT RAIDING THE RAGS 'N' MAGS AISLE.

WAAA!

I BUILT CHECKLISTS; BECAME A **COMPLETIST.**

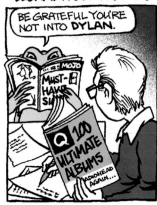

BE GRATEFUL YOU'RE NOT INTO **DYLAN.**

Q 100 ULTIMATE ALBUMS

INSTEAD OF WORKING, I SPENT HOURS, DAYS, SURFING FOR OBSCURE HUNGARIAN FLICKS FROM THE SIXTIES.

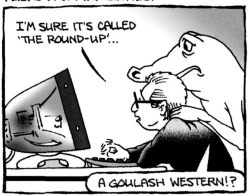

I'M SURE IT'S CALLED 'THE ROUND-UP'...

A GOULASH WESTERN!?

I FOUND MYSELF **REGRESSING,** REDISCOVERING STUFF I LAPPED UP IN MY YOUTH.

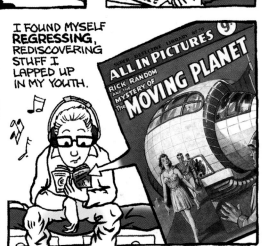

ALL IN PICTURES

RICK RANDOM AND THE MYSTERY OF The **MOVING PLANET**

(A LOT OF IT SEEMED TO BE WAR AND HIGH ADVENTURE.)

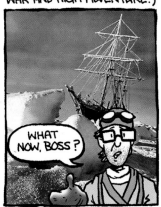

WHAT NOW, BOSS?

I COLLECTED LIBRARIES OF CLOBBER IT WOULD TAKE ME **DECADES** TO GET THROUGH...

BUT POSSESSION IS 9/10ths OF THE **COMFORT ZONE** ...

AND THE HEADPHONES WERE RARELY OFF.

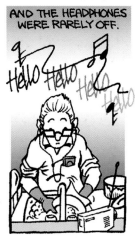

Hello Hello Hello Hello

97

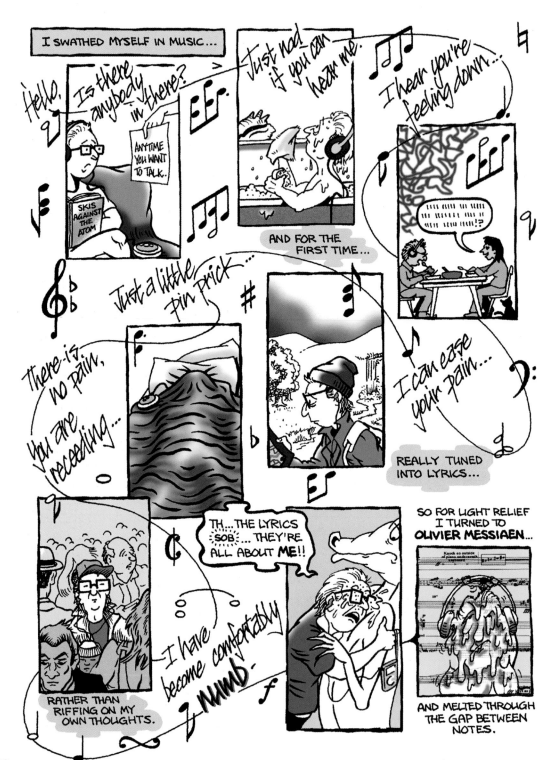

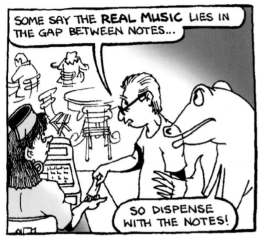

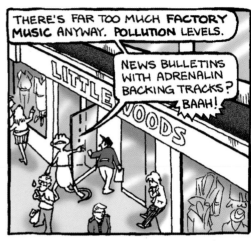

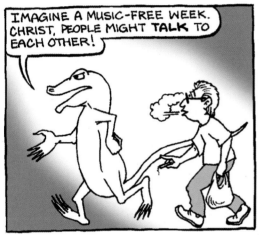

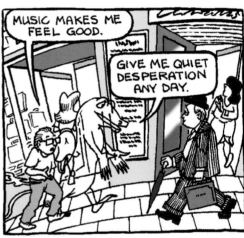

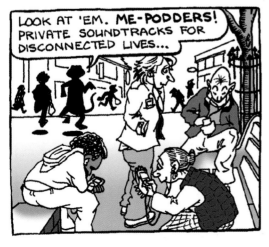

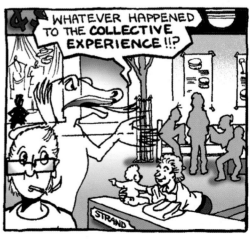

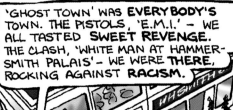

'GHOST TOWN' WAS **EVERYBODY'S** TOWN. THE PISTOLS, 'E.M.I.' – WE ALL TASTED **SWEET REVENGE**. THE CLASH, 'WHITE MAN AT HAMMER-SMITH PALAIS' – WE WERE **THERE**, ROCKING AGAINST **RACISM**.

YOU'RE STUCK IN A ROSE-TINTED **TIMEWARP**, PAL.

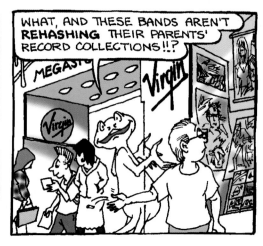

WHAT, AND THESE BANDS AREN'T **REHASHING** THEIR PARENTS' RECORD COLLECTIONS!!?

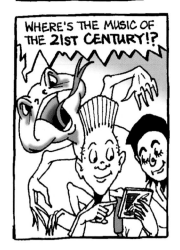

WHERE'S THE MUSIC OF THE 21ST CENTURY!?

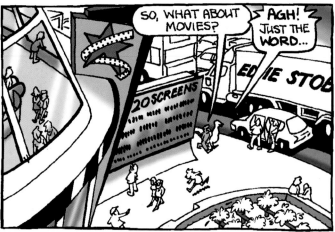

SO, WHAT ABOUT MOVIES?

AGH! JUST THE WORD...

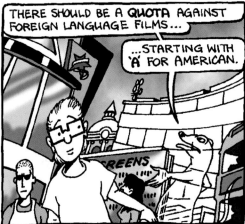

THERE SHOULD BE A **QUOTA** AGAINST FOREIGN LANGUAGE FILMS...

...STARTING WITH 'A' FOR AMERICAN.

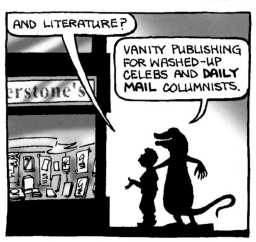

AND LITERATURE?

VANITY PUBLISHING FOR WASHED-UP CELEBS AND **DAILY MAIL** COLUMNISTS.

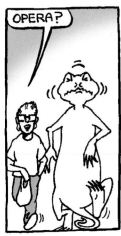

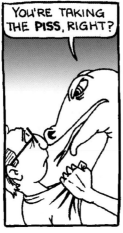

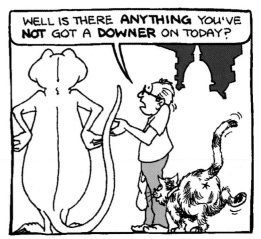

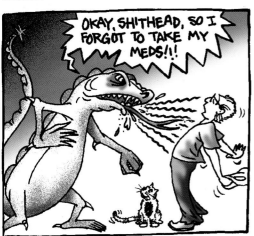

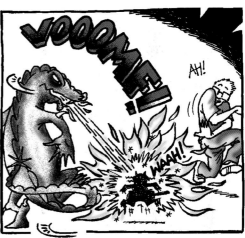

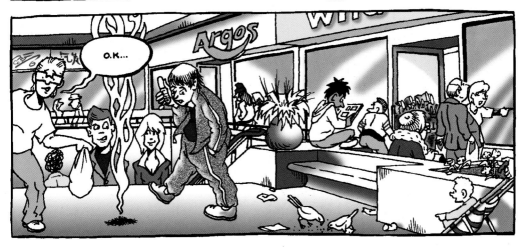

AND I HAD ANOTHER NEW COMPULSION — DARK, DANGEROUS, POTENTIALLY **BLINDING**.

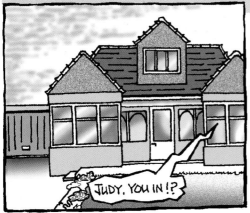

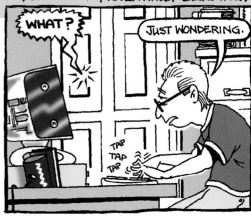

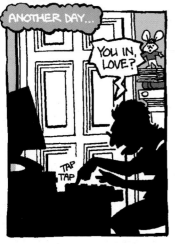

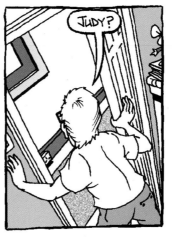

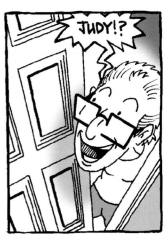

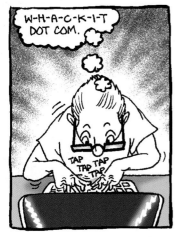

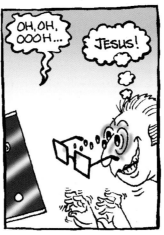

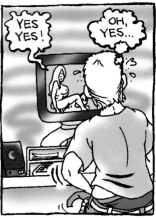

WHAT CAN I TELL YOU?

ACCORDING TO THE LITERATURE, MY LIBIDO SHOULD HAVE VACATED THE PREMISES.

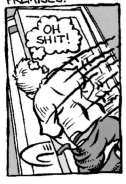

OH SHIT!

YET I WANTED TO JUMP JUDY EVERY NANOSECOND OF THE DAY.

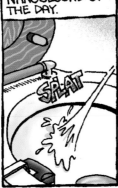

SPLAT

I COULDN'T WALK DOWN THE STREET WITHOUT X-RAYING EVERY BOUNCING BOSSOM AND BUM.

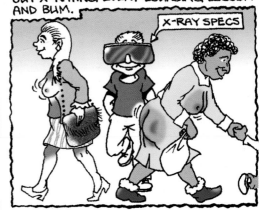

X-RAY SPECS

AT HOME, I COULDN'T OPEN **SAFARI** WITHOUT HITTING THE BOOKMARK.

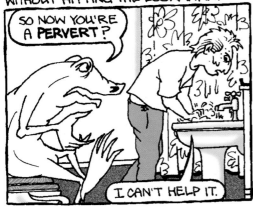

SO NOW YOU'RE A **PERVERT**?

I CAN'T HELP IT.

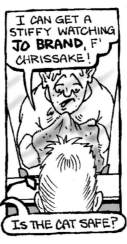

I CAN GET A STIFFY WATCHING **JO BRAND**, F' CHRISSAKE!

IS THE CAT SAFE?

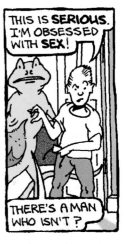

THIS IS **SERIOUS**. I'M OBSESSED WITH **SEX**!

THERE'S A MAN WHO ISN'T?

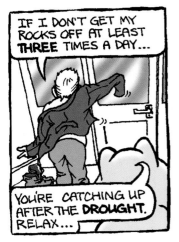

IF I DON'T GET MY ROCKS OFF AT LEAST **THREE** TIMES A DAY...

YOU'RE CATCHING UP AFTER THE **DROUGHT**. RELAX...

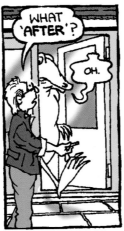

WHAT 'AFTER'?

OH.

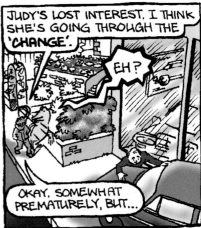

JUDY'S LOST INTEREST. I THINK SHE'S GOING THROUGH THE 'CHANGE'.

EH?

OKAY, SOMEWHAT PREMATURELY, BUT...

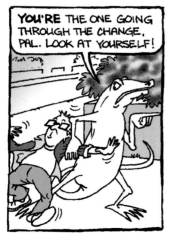

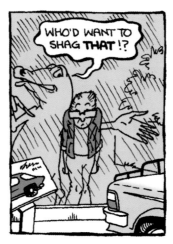

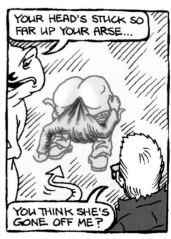

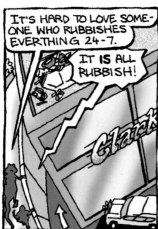

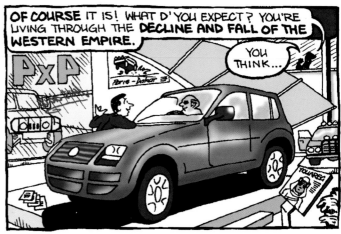

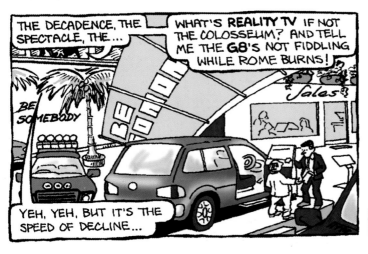

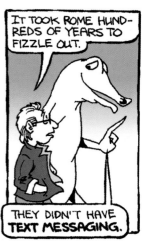

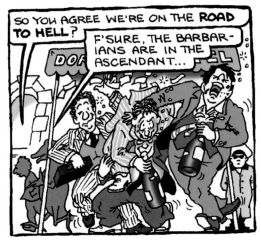

SO YOU AGREE WE'RE ON THE **ROAD TO HELL**?

F'SURE, THE BARBARIANS ARE IN THE ASCENDANT...

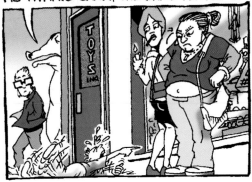

BUT THAT'S NO REASON TO BE SUCH A **GODDAMN MISERY**. OKAY, CIVILISATION'S GURGLING DOWN THE U-BEND, BUT EVEN AS TITANIC SANK, THE BAND **PLAYED ON**.

YOU NEED TO **RISE ABOVE** THE DEBACLE, LAUGH AT ITS **INSANITY**. HELL, IF I HAD YOUR SKILLS, I'D BE HAVING A **FIELD DAY**.

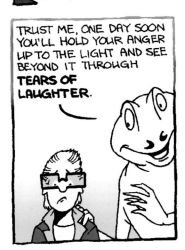

JUST MAKES ME FUCKIN' **ANGRY**.

NAAR. THE BIG BAD WORLD'S SIMPLY YOUR **WHIPPING BOY**. I'M AFRAID THE BUTT OF YOUR RAGE LIES MUCH DEEPER.

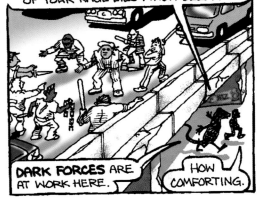

DARK FORCES ARE AT WORK HERE.

HOW COMFORTING.

TRUST ME, ONE DAY SOON YOU'LL HOLD YOUR ANGER UP TO THE LIGHT AND SEE BEYOND IT THROUGH **TEARS OF LAUGHTER**.

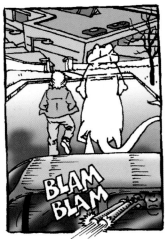

BLAM BLAM

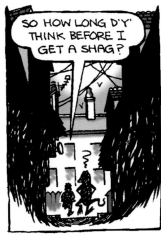

SO HOW LONG D'Y' THINK BEFORE I GET A SHAG?

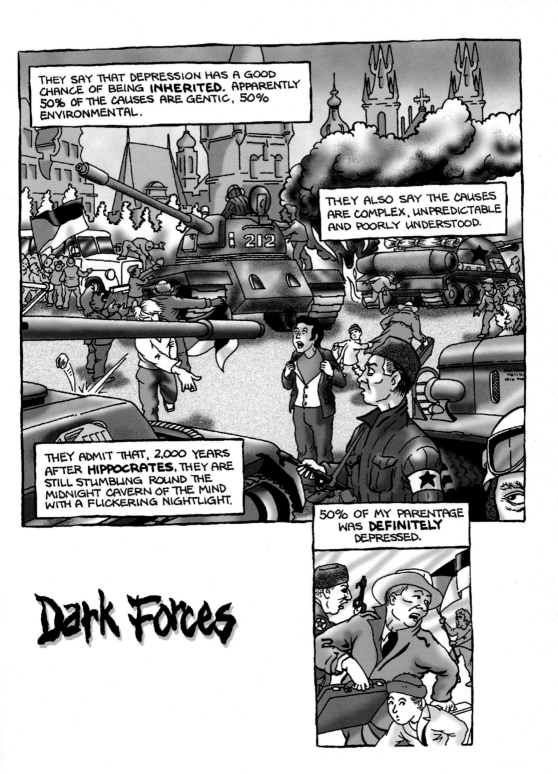

MUCH AS I LOVED HER, MY MOTHER WAS A MISERY. THE SADNESS THAT CONSUMED HER WAS NEVER EXPRESSED, NOT TO A DOCTOR OR PRIEST, NOT EVEN TO MY FATHER.

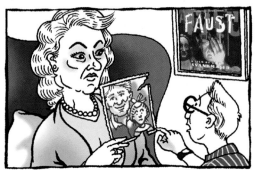

THAT'S NOT QUITE TRUE. THE PAIN WAS ETCHED DEEP IN HER FACE, BUT MAYBE ONLY I COULD READ THE RUNES. I INHERITED HER MELANCHOLIC MOUTH.

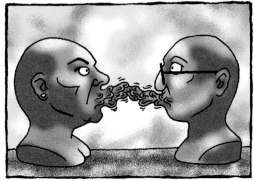

WHAT WE KNOW ABOUT MY MOTHER BEGINS THE DAY SHE MET MY FATHER AT A DINNER-DANCE IN THE CATTERICK GARRISON'S SERGEANTS MESS. THE GIRLS WERE BUSSED IN FROM A LOCAL WOMEN'S COLLEGE.

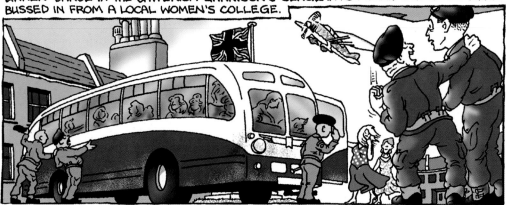

DAD WAS ANOTHER SAD SACK, BORN AND RAISED IN COMMERCIAL HOTELS RUN BY HIS MOTHER. HIS FATHER WAS A CHEF SOMEWHERE OR OTHER.

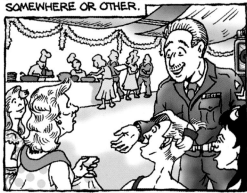

THE ARMY HAD BECOME HIS FAMILY, BUT HE TALKED ABOUT HIS ITINERATE CHILDHOOD, MOVING TOWN EVERY FEW YEARS, SLEEPING IN EMPTY GUEST ROOMS, NEVER IN THE SAME BED LONGER THAN A WEEK.

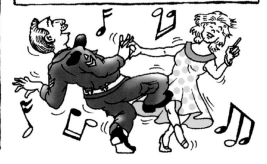

MY MUM WAS A CLOSED BOOK, BUCKLED AND LOCKED. BUT BEFORE HE DIED, I PRIZED FRAGMENTS OF HER STORY OUT OF THE ONLY GRANDPARENT I KNEW, HER FATHER, MIKLÓS.

SHE WAS A CHILD REFUGEE, FLEEING CZECHOSLOVAKIA WITH MIKLÓS WHEN THE **COLD WAR** WAS BELOW FREEZING FOR THE CZECHS.

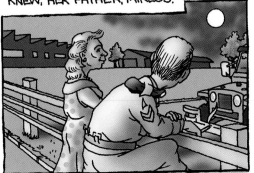

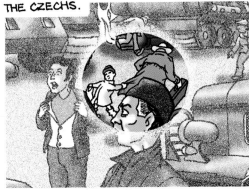

I WAS AN ENGINEER AT A HYDRO PLANT IN THE JESENIKY MOUNTAINS.

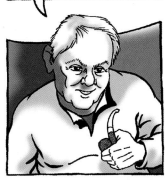

THE RUSSIANS BEGAN BUILDING SOMETHING **BIG** UP THERE. HOLLOWED OUT A MOUNTAIN, LAID A RAILWAY.

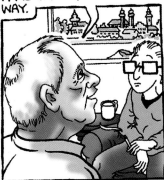

IT WAS A NUCLEAR DEFENCE SITE FOR A HUGE LASER CANNON; A PROTOTYPE 'BIG BERTHA' OF THE ATOMIC AGE. CRAZY!

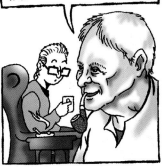

"YOU CAN'T DISPERSE THAT MUCH EARTH WITHOUT EVERY HILL FARMER KNOWS IT. BUT THE MOUNTAINS WERE A RESTRICTED ZONE...

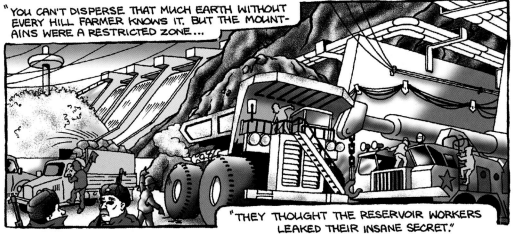

"THEY THOUGHT THE RESERVOIR WORKERS LEAKED THEIR INSANE SECRET."

"THEY STARTED ARRESTING THE CZECHS, BUT WE HAD A HOLIDAY BOOKED. WE ESCAPED FROM YUGOSLAVIA, JUST YOUR MOTHER AND ME."

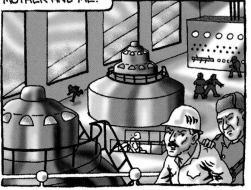

"(IF A FAMILY WENT TO THE SEA, ONE PARENT HAD TO STAY BEHIND AS HOSTAGE TO MAKE SURE THEY RETURNED.)"

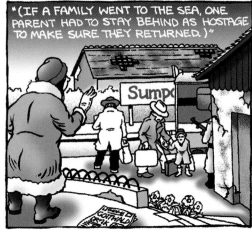

ANA, YOUR GRANDMA, AGREED WE MUST GO. WE THOUGHT WE COULD GET HER OUT LATER, BUT THE StB* WATCHED HER LIKE HAWKS.

IMMIGRAT... ...NTROL PORT AUT... ...OVER

* SECRET POLICE

SHE DIED BEFORE **GLASNOST**, BEFORE WE COULD BE A FAMILY AGAIN.

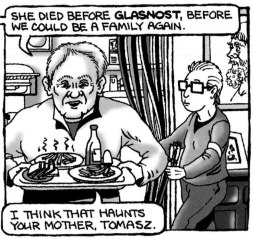

I THINK THAT HAUNTS YOUR MOTHER, TOMASZ.

MY FOLKS WERE TWO **LOST SOULS** THAT COLLIDED, FUSED AND WERE BORN AGAIN INTO THE FAMILY OF THE BRITISH ARMY.

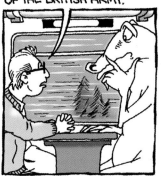

THEY HAD A GREAT LIFE TOGETHER - TRAVELLED THE WORLD, LIVED IN EXOTIC PLACES...

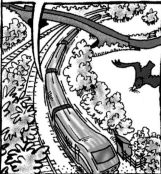

...AND HAD ONE CHILD, WHO SPENT MOST OF THAT TIME IN A BOARDING SCHOOL.

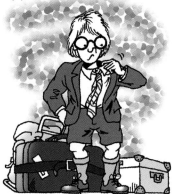

110

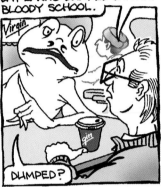

ODDLY ENOUGH I HAVE COMPLETE AMNESIA ABOUT EVERYTHING BEFORE THE DAY I WAS DUMPED IN THAT BLOODY SCHOOL.

DUMPED?

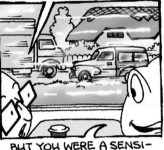

OKAY, THEY THOUGHT THEY WERE DOING THE RIGHT THING – STABLE ENVIRONMENT, GOOD EDUCATION...

BUT YOU WERE A SENSITIVE PETAL, NEEDED YOUR MUMMY...

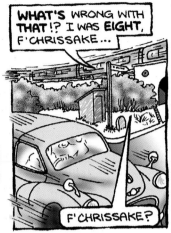

WHAT'S WRONG WITH THAT!? I WAS EIGHT, F'CHRISSAKE...

F'CHRISSAKE?

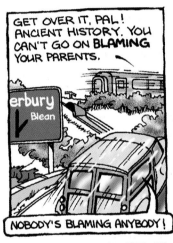

GET OVER IT, PAL! ANCIENT HISTORY. YOU CAN'T GO ON BLAMING YOUR PARENTS.

erbury
Blean

NOBODY'S BLAMING ANYBODY!

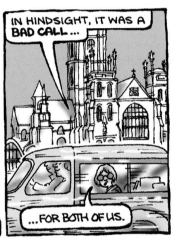

IN HINDSIGHT, IT WAS A BAD CALL...

...FOR BOTH OF US.

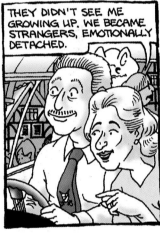

THEY DIDN'T SEE ME GROWING UP. WE BECAME STRANGERS, EMOTIONALLY DETACHED.

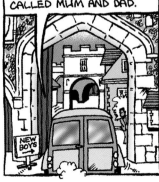

HOME WAS THE SCHOOL, THIS MEDIEVAL CLOISTER. NOW AND THEN I VISITED SOME ACQUAINTANCES CALLED MUM AND DAD.

NEW BOYS

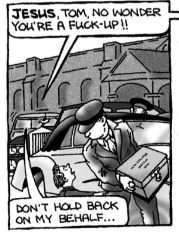

JESUS, TOM, NO WONDER YOU'RE A FUCK-UP!!

DON'T HOLD BACK ON MY BEHALF...

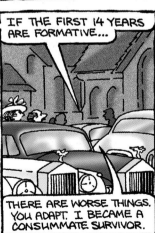

IF THE FIRST 14 YEARS ARE FORMATIVE...

THERE ARE WORSE THINGS. YOU ADAPT. I BECAME A CONSUMMATE SURVIVOR.

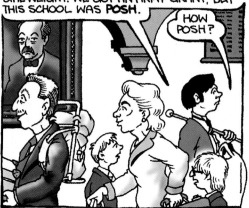

MY FOLKS WERE HITTING ABOVE THEIR FINANCIAL WEIGHT. WE GOT AN ARMY GRANT, BUT THIS SCHOOL WAS **POSH.**

HOW POSH?

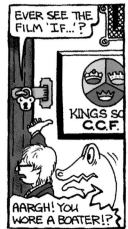

EVER SEE THE FILM 'IF...'?

KINGS SC C.C.F.

AARGH! YOU WORE A BOATER!?

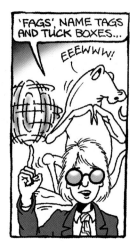

'FAGS', NAME TAGS AND TUCK BOXES...

EEEWWW!

THERE WERE AFRICAN PRINCES AND HEIRS TO COUNTRY PILES IN MY CLASS, AND ANOTHER FREEMAN OF HARDY AND WILLIS FAME.

Future...

MP   DUKE   DICTATOR   JUDGE

BANKER   CEO   GENERAL

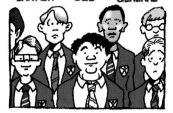

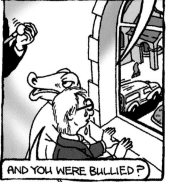

SPOILT BUGGERS, MOST OF 'EM THICKER THAN THEIR INHERITANCE PORTFOLIOS.

AND YOU WERE BULLIED?

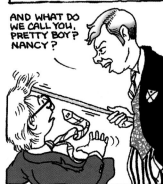

BY THEM, PSYCHOLOGICALLY. THEY LEFT BEATINGS TO THE STAFF.

AND WHAT DO WE CALL YOU, PRETTY BOY? NANCY?

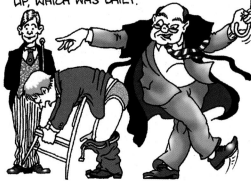

PLEBBY KIDS LIKE ME WERE THE FALL-GUYS. WE GOT IT IN THE NECK (OR ON THE BUM) WHEN THE RICH KIDS SCREWED UP, WHICH WAS DAILY.

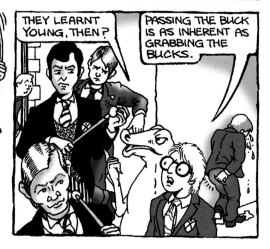

THEY LEARNT YOUNG, THEN?

PASSING THE BUCK IS AS INHERENT AS GRABBING THE BUCKS.

112

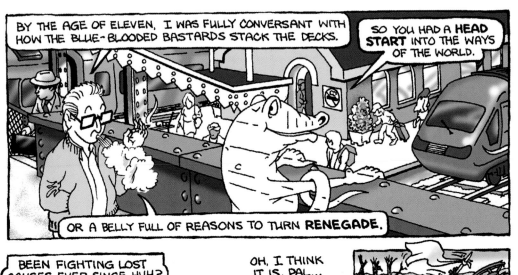

BY THE AGE OF ELEVEN, I WAS FULLY CONVERSANT WITH HOW THE BLUE-BLOODED BASTARDS STACK THE DECKS.

SO YOU HAD A **HEAD START** INTO THE WAYS OF THE WORLD.

OR A BELLY FULL OF REASONS TO TURN **RENEGADE**.

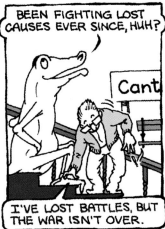

BEEN FIGHTING LOST CAUSES EVER SINCE, HUH?

I'VE LOST BATTLES, BUT THE WAR ISN'T OVER.

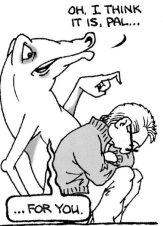

OH, I THINK IT IS, PAL...

... FOR YOU.

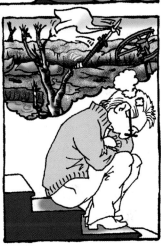

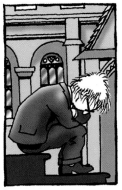

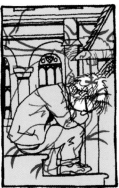

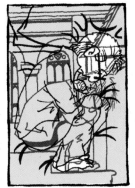

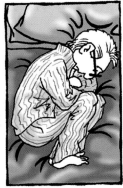

RETURNING FROM CHINA, IT WAS HARD TO DISAPPEAR. EVERYBODY WANTED TO HEAR OUR TALES. WHILE JUDY DID THE ROUNDS AND MADE APOLOGIES, I HID UNDER THE DUVET, WISHING THE WORLD WOULD DISAPPEAR UP ITS OWN BLACK HOLE.

THE RUG HAD BEEN PULLED FROM UNDER MY VERY BEING, FOLLOWED BY THE FLOORBOARDS, JOISTS AND FOUNDATIONS.

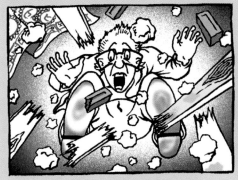

I WAS A WASTE OF SPACE, **USELESS**, A SPAZZER, **ME**, WHO HAD CROSSED THE SAHARA **WITHOUT** A SWISS ARMY KNIFE AND COULD SOLVE A RUBIK'S CUBE IN **34** SECONDS.

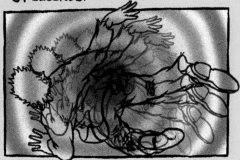

I WAS TRAPPED IN A MORBID LABYRINTH WITH A MONSTER WHO HAD TURNED AGAINST ME; AN OLD, OLD FRIEND WHO NOW TERRIFIED ME.

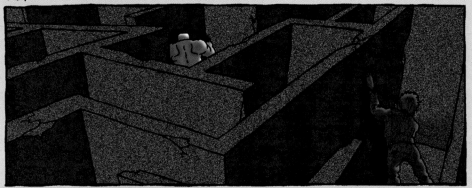

WE STALKED EACH OTHER FOR WEEKS. TIMES WHEN I THOUGHT WE CAME FACE TO FACE WERE MORE LIKELY A TRICK OF THE LIGHT...

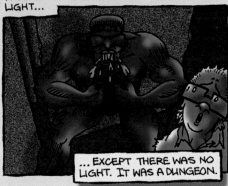

...EXCEPT THERE WAS NO LIGHT. IT WAS A DUNGEON.

IN MOMENTS OF RESPITE I MOURNED MY DEARLY DEPARTED SELF, DROWNING IN A QUAGMIRE OF **MELANCHOLY**; AN OLD WORD BUT A GOOD WORD, RARELY USED.

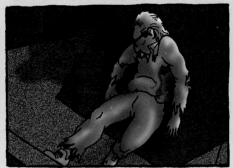

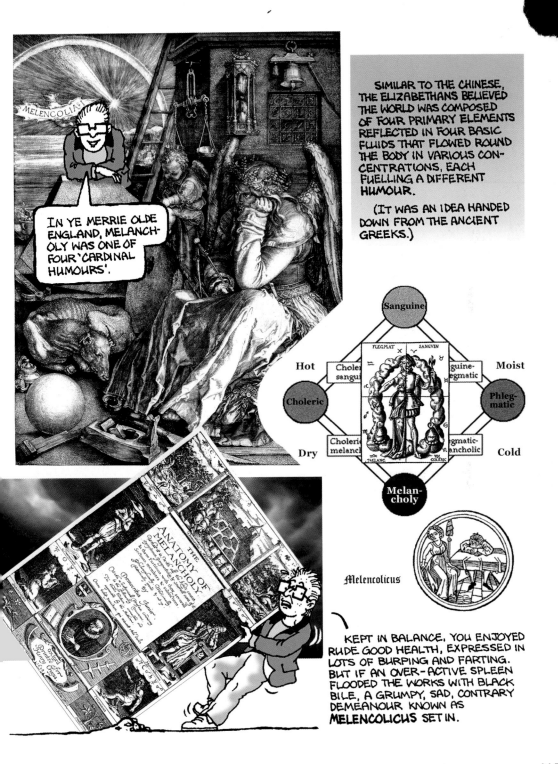

SIMILAR TO THE CHINESE, THE ELIZABETHANS BELIEVED THE WORLD WAS COMPOSED OF FOUR PRIMARY ELEMENTS REFLECTED IN FOUR BASIC FLUIDS THAT FLOWED ROUND THE BODY IN VARIOUS CONCENTRATIONS, EACH FUELLING A DIFFERENT HUMOUR.

(IT WAS AN IDEA HANDED DOWN FROM THE ANCIENT GREEKS.)

IN YE MERRIE OLDE ENGLAND, MELANCHOLY WAS ONE OF FOUR 'CARDINAL HUMOURS'.

KEPT IN BALANCE, YOU ENJOYED RUDE GOOD HEALTH, EXPRESSED IN LOTS OF BURPING AND FARTING. BUT IF AN OVER-ACTIVE SPLEEN FLOODED THE WORKS WITH BLACK BILE, A GRUMPY, SAD, CONTRARY DEMEANOUR KNOWN AS **MELENCOLICUS** SET IN.

115

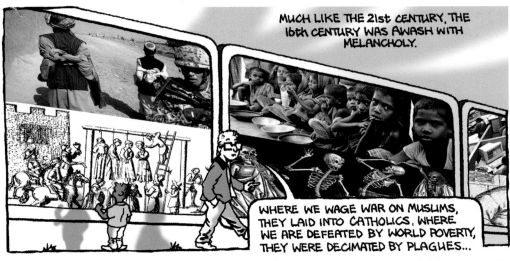

MUCH LIKE THE 21st CENTURY, THE 16th CENTURY WAS AWASH WITH MELANCHOLY.

WHERE WE WAGE WAR ON MUSLIMS, THEY LAID INTO CATHOLICS, WHERE WE ARE DEFEATED BY WORLD POVERTY, THEY WERE DECIMATED BY PLAGUES...

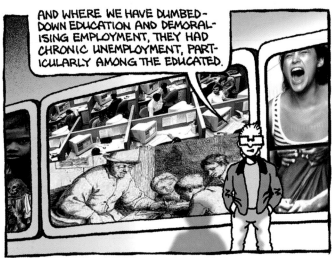

AND WHERE WE HAVE DUMBED-DOWN EDUCATION AND DEMORAL-ISING EMPLOYMENT, THEY HAD CHRONIC UNEMPLOYMENT, PART-ICULARLY AMONG THE EDUCATED.

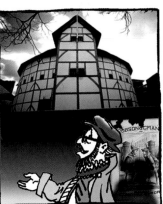

THEN THERE WAS CRAP WEATHER, CRAP DIETS AND A CRAP LOVE LIFE. NOTHING CHANGES...

THEN AS NOW, MELANCHOLY WAS SO PREVALENT IT WAS POSITIVELY FASHIONABLE. PERFECTLY HAPPY CHAPPIES WOULD FEIGN MELANCHOLY HOPING IT ENDOWED THEM WITH THE GRAVITAS OF A **HAMLET** (A MAN WITH MORE VOICES ZAPPING ROUND HIS HEAD THAN A CALL CENTRE).
STALKING THE STREETS WEARING A BLACK HAT AND A FACE LIKE THE BACK END OF A NIGHT SOIL CART MEANT YOU WERE EITHER A DEEPLY TROUBLED INTELLECTUAL OR A DEEPLY TROUBLED **TOSSER.**

ENTER THE STEREOTYPE OF THE TORMENTED POET, ABOUT THE ONLY PEOPLE TODAY WHO AREN'T SHY TO USE 'MELANCHOLY' IN PUBLIC.

WHAT A PIECE OF WORK IS A MAN; ANGRY, CONFUSED, UP-TIGHT, MISERABLE...

IF THE HUMOURS ARE NOW HISTORY, THE ELIZABETHANS GAVE US ONE NOTION THAT REFUSES TO FADE. AS DR. TWITCH SO ELOQUENTLY PUT IT...

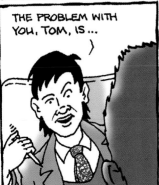

THE PROBLEM WITH YOU, TOM, IS...

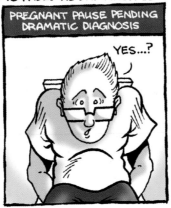

PREGNANT PAUSE PENDING DRAMATIC DIAGNOSIS

YES...?

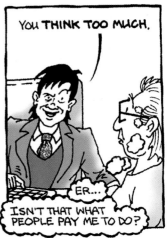

YOU **THINK TOO MUCH.**

ER...

ISN'T THAT WHAT PEOPLE PAY ME TO DO?

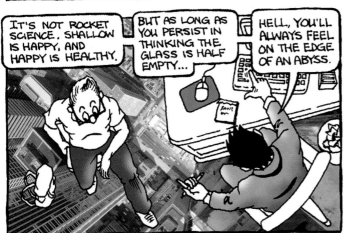

IT'S NOT ROCKET SCIENCE. SHALLOW IS HAPPY, AND HAPPY IS HEALTHY.

BUT AS LONG AS YOU PERSIST IN THINKING THE GLASS IS HALF EMPTY...

HELL, YOU'LL ALWAYS FEEL ON THE EDGE OF AN ABYSS.

400 YEARS ON, WE ARE STILL PEDDLING THE IDEA THAT THE ANTIDOTE TO MELANCHOLY IS SIMPLY TO TURN YOUR PERCEPTION OF **REALITY** ON ITS HEAD.

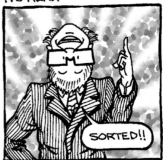

SORTED!!

POSITIVE THINKING HAS HIT FETISH LEVELS IN THE WEST. HUMAN CAPITAL CONSULTANTS, SELF HELP GURUS, COGNITIVE BEHAVIOURAL THERAPISTS, EVEN CHECK-OUT GIRLS...

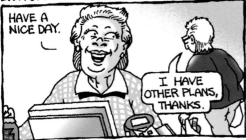

HAVE A NICE DAY.

I HAVE OTHER PLANS, THANKS.

IT WAS HARD TO TURN A CORNER WITHOUT CRASHING INTO THE MANTRA, "THE GLASS IS HALF FULL, THE GLASS IS HALF..."

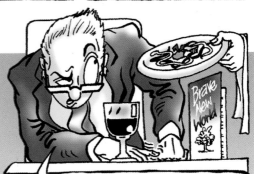

WAS I THINKING TOO MUCH TO WONDER WHY WE ARE SO OBSESSED? LIKE HOW COME NO-BODY'S UP IN ARMS ABOUT THE RIP-OFF RESTAURANT WHERE THE MEASURE SERVED IS ALWAYS SO MEANLY BORDERLINE?!!?

ONE THING THE ELIZABETHANS WERE
RIGHT ABOUT, DEPRESSION IS A
DISEASE OF THE IMAGINATION. WITNESS...

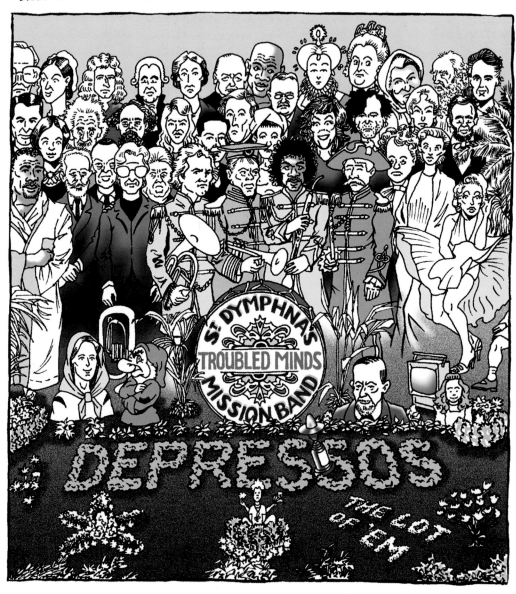

LEFT TO RIGHT FROM TOP:

CHARLES SCHULTZ, FLORENCE NIGHTINGALE, ISSAC NEWTON, JAMES WATT, VIRGINIA WOOLF, WINSTON CHURCHILL, FRANK
BRUNO, ELIZABETH I, CATHERINE THE GREAT, INDIRA GANDHI, LEO TOLSTOY, MARIE CURIE, CARY GRANT, CHARLOTTE
BRONTE, ALBERT EINSTEIN, CHARLES DICKENS, SYLVIA PLATH, COLE PORTER, HANS CHRISTIAN ANDERSON, NIJINSKY,
THEODORE ROOSEVELT, KAREN CARPENTER, TIM BURTON, JMW TURNER, ABRAHAM LINCOLN, MIKE TYSON, PETER
TCHAIKOVSKY, SERGEI RACHMANINOFF, ERIC CLAPTON, BRIAN WILSON, LUDWIG VAN BEETHOVEN, DAVID BOWIE, JIM HENDRIX,
EDWARD ELGAR, DYLAN THOMAS, JUDY GARLAND, MARILYN MONROE, SAINT DYMPHNA, GRUMPY, SIGMUND FREUD AND
LENA ZAVARONI.

ST. DYMPHNA: PATRON SAINT OF FRUITCAKES

IT CROSSED MY MIND TO TRY A MEDIEVAL REMEDY FOR MY 'MELENCOLICUS', EXCEPT...

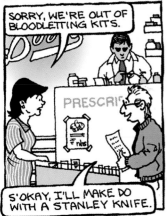

SORRY, WE'RE OUT OF BLOODLETTING KITS.

PRESCRI...

S'OKAY, I'LL MAKE DO WITH A STANLEY KNIFE.

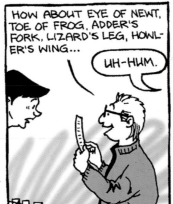

HOW ABOUT EYE OF NEWT, TOE OF FROG, ADDER'S FORK, LIZARD'S LEG, HOWLER'S WING...

UH-HUM.

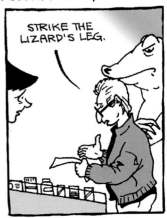

STRIKE THE LIZARD'S LEG.

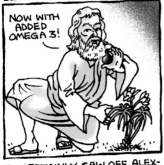

AS ENDORSED BY HIPPOCRATES, HELLEBORE WAS SUPPOSED TO BE AN ALL-TIME FAVOURITE.

NOW WITH ADDED OMEGA 3!

IT CERTAINLY SAW OFF ALEXANDER THE GREAT'S DEPRESSIONS... IT KILLED HIM.

THERE HAD TO BE A VARIETY OF HELEBORE THAT WASN'T LETHAL, BUT I COULDN'T TELL A PANSY FROM A PETUNIA. AT MY LOCAL GARDEN CENTRE THEY CONVINCED ME I'D FEEL A LOT BETTER IF I SETTLED FOR 100 SQ.MTRS. OF DECKING.

MEANTIME, BACK IN THE DUNGEON, I HAD MORE CHANCE OF GOLD IN THE WOMEN'S SHOT PUT THAN OF CONJOURING A SINGLE POSITIVE THOUGHT.

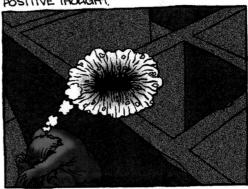

I WAS THINKING ALRIGHT, THINKING ABOUT **EVERYTHING**, DELIBERATING ON DELIBERATIONS AND THE ANGLES OF EACH DELIBERATION, THINKING UNTIL I'D THOUGHT MYSELF INTO OBLIVION.

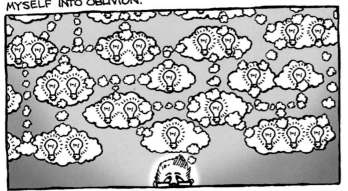

SLEEP WAS ABOUT THE ONLY POSITIVE THING GOING FOR ME RIGHT THEN.

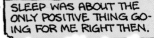

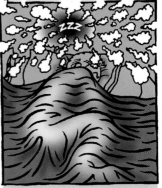

TOO OFTEN IT ELUDED ME.

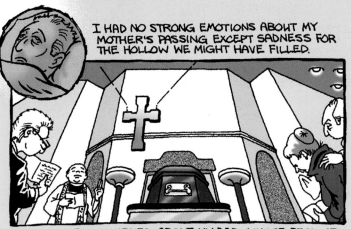

I HAD NO STRONG EMOTIONS ABOUT MY MOTHER'S PASSING EXCEPT SADNESS FOR THE HOLLOW WE MIGHT HAVE FILLED.

I WAS MORE CONCERNED ABOUT MY DAD, WHOSE PEAK OF CULINARY SUCCESS WAS A RUNNY OMELETTE BACK IN 2001.

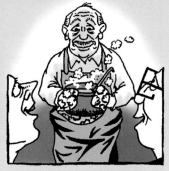

(HE ROSE TO THE CHALLENGE, LEARNED TO LOOK AFTER HIMSELF AND SERVED GAZPACHO AND A FIREY GOULASH ON OUR LAST VISIT.)

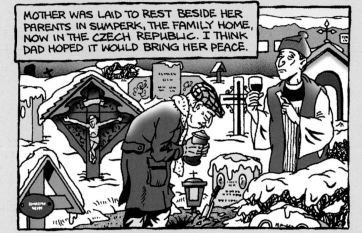

MOTHER WAS LAID TO REST BESIDE HER PARENTS IN SUMPERK, THE FAMILY HOME, NOW IN THE CZECH REPUBLIC. I THINK DAD HOPED IT WOULD BRING HER PEACE.

FOUR YEARS LATER, JUDY AND I MADE THE PILGRIMAGE.

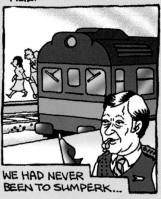

WE HAD NEVER BEEN TO SUMPERK...

BUT I WAS SOMEHOW FAMILIAR WITH THE LIE OF THE TOWN. THE COMMIES HAD DONE A JOB ON THE PLACE, YET IT FELT LIKE HOME.

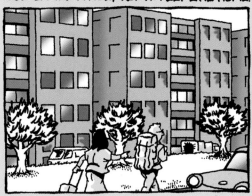

AND I KNEW WHICH CHURCH WAS THEIRS WITHOUT BEING SHOWN. I HAD SOME NOTION MUM WAS CHRISTENED THERE.

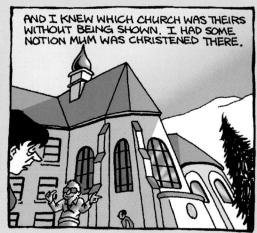

BUT SHE WAS NO LONGER BURIED THERE. THE PAYMENTS HAD LAPSED, DAD HAD MOVED AND NOTIFICATION WENT ASTRAY.

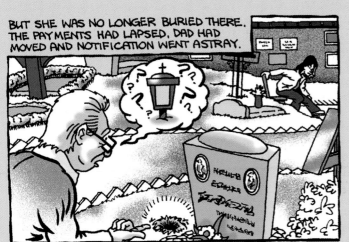

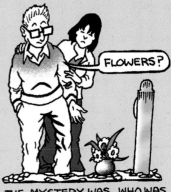

FLOWERS?

THE MYSTERY WAS, WHO WAS PAYING FOR MY GRAND PARENTS' PLOT?

BETWEEN THE CHURCH AND TOWN HALL, EVERYTHING GOT LOST IN TRANSLATION, PARTICULARLY MOTHER'S URN.

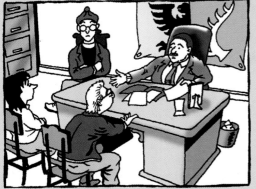

NOT EVEN **DISTANT** RELATIVES COULD BE TRACED, BUT WE TRACKED DOWN GRANNY ANA'S OLDEST FRIEND.

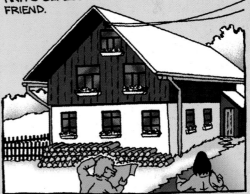

THROUGH HER SON, SHE QUIETLY WARDED US OFF. "SOME THINGS ARE BEST TO NOT DISTURB," HE SAID.

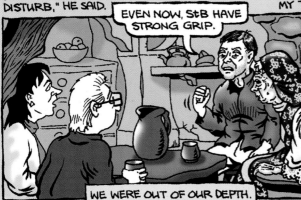

EVEN NOW, StB HAVE STRONG GRIP.

WE WERE OUT OF OUR DEPTH.

THE JOURNEY HOME WAS A DAZE. FLOODS OF CASCADING THOUGHTS HAMMERED AT MY TEMPLES.

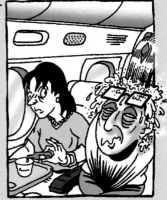

CAST ASHES TO THE WIND, A LANDMARK REMAINS TO ANCHOR MEMORIES – A HILLTOP, A BAY...

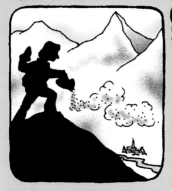

BUT MY MOTHER WAS JUST KICKING AROUND SUMPERK SOMEWHERE, MAYBE A DOORSTOP, MAYBE A WEIGHT.

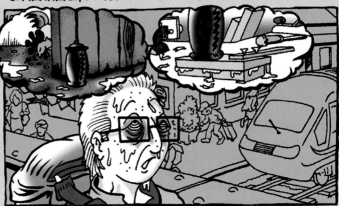

TOM!!

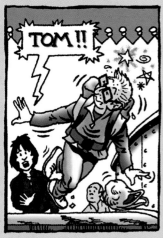

I COLLAPSED AT THE STATION AND BRIEFLY BLACKED OUT.

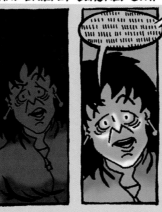

... AND WE'LL CONTACT THE EMBASSY, HIRE A TRANSLATOR...

I WOULDN'T BOTHER. IT'S PAR FOR THE COURSE WITH MY FAMILY.

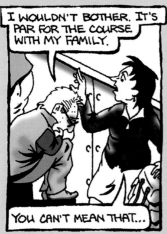

YOU CAN'T MEAN THAT...

IT'LL TROUBLE YOU FOREVER.

HMM... GOT THE TICKETS?

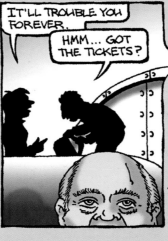

DELIBERATIONS ON DELIBERATIONS...

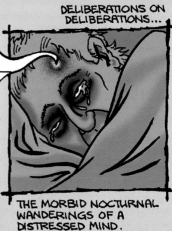

THE MORBID NOCTURNAL WANDERINGS OF A DISTRESSED MIND.

SOMETIMES I JUST LAY THERE WONDERING IF I SHOULD WORRY THAT MY CHEST HAD TURNED INTO TECTONIC PLATES.

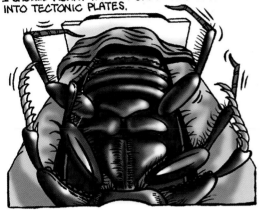

NOW AND AGAIN I VENTURED OUT TO SATISFY MY CONSUMER COMPULSIONS, TERRIFIED SOMEBODY MIGHT RECOGNISE ME.

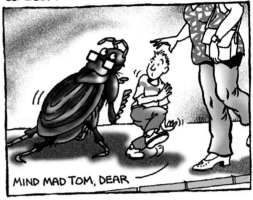

MIND MAD TOM, DEAR

FOR THREE MONTHS I MANAGED TO AVOID ALL CONTACT WITH FAMILIAR FACES.

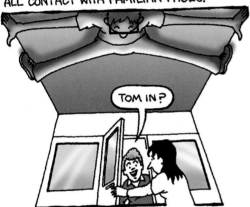

TOM IN?

THE RUMOUR MILL STARTED CHURNING. IN THE GUISE OF SUPPORT, CALLS, CARDS AND EMAILS CAME LOOKING FOR GRIST.

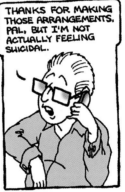

THANKS FOR MAKING THOSE ARRANGEMENTS, PAL, BUT I'M NOT ACTUALLY FEELING SUICIDAL.

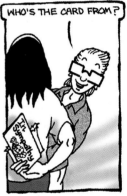

WHO'S THE CARD FROM?

I SENSED A SUDDEN RUSH OF VOLUNTEERS EAGER TO STAFF THE SAMARITANS' LINE.

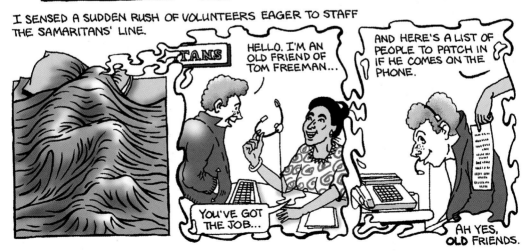

HELLO. I'M AN OLD FRIEND OF TOM FREEMAN...

AND HERE'S A LIST OF PEOPLE TO PATCH IN IF HE COMES ON THE PHONE.

YOU'VE GOT THE JOB...

AH YES, OLD FRIENDS.

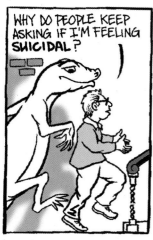

WHY DO PEOPLE KEEP ASKING IF I'M FEELING **SUICIDAL**?

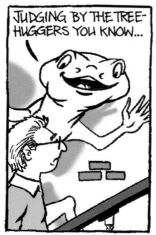

JUDGING BY THE TREE-HUGGERS YOU KNOW...

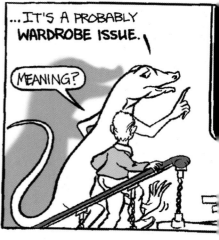

...IT'S A PROBABLY **WARDROBE ISSUE**.

MEANING?

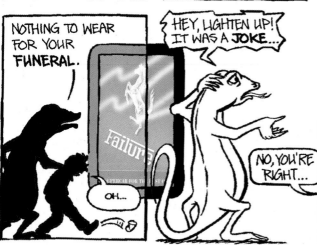

NOTHING TO WEAR FOR YOUR **FUNERAL**.

Failure

OH...

HEY, LIGHTEN UP! IT WAS A **JOKE**...

NO, YOU'RE RIGHT...

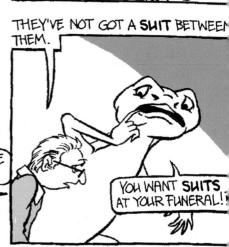

THEY'VE NOT GOT A **SUIT** BETWEEN THEM.

YOU WANT **SUITS** AT YOUR FUNERAL!?

WHAT I WANT IS ORSON WELLES READING, JOE STRUMMER SINGING, AND THE CAST OF **SUPERVIXENS** AS PALL BEARERS.

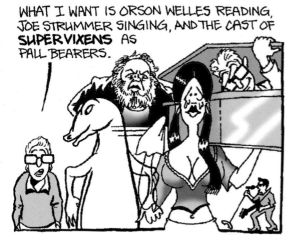

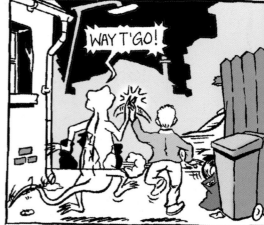

WAY T'GO!

124

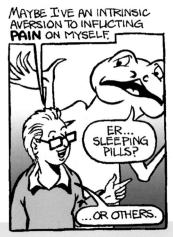

Panel 1: ANYROAD, I'VE NEVER BEEN BIG ON SUICIDE.

MAYBE YOU'VE NEVER HIT **ROCK BOTTOM**?

Panel 2: MAYBE I'VE AN INTRINSIC AVERSION TO INFLICTING **PAIN** ON MYSELF.

ER... SLEEPING PILLS?

...OR OTHERS.

Panel 3: WE TALKING **EMOTIONAL**?

WHATEVER. PAIN IS PAIN.

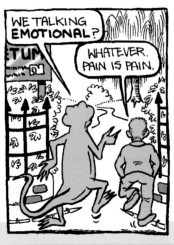

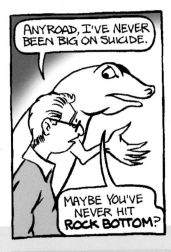

ONCE I NEARLY PUT A KID'S EYE OUT. GEORGE BUTCHER AND MYSELF WERE CLEARING THE SCHOOL ALLOTMENT, BUILDING A COMPOST HEAP.

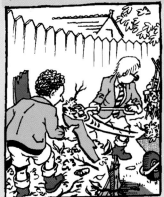

BUTCHER WAS FANNYING AROUND ON THE HEAP.

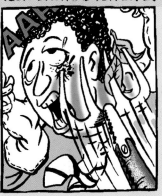

I SPEARED HIM JUST UNDER THE LEFT EYE. SCARRED THE POOR BASTARD FOR **LIFE**.

AAL

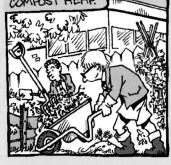

STILL **IRKS** ME, THAT DOES.

OH PLEASE!

AND **THAT'S** WHY YOU DON'T WAKE UP EVERY MORNING WITH THE **OVERWHELMING DESIRE** TO TOP YOURSELF!?

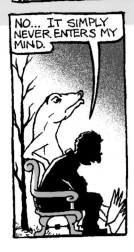

NO... IT SIMPLY NEVER ENTERS MY MIND.

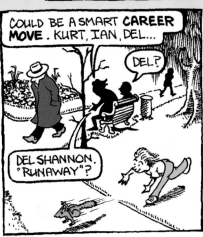

COULD BE A SMART **CAREER MOVE**. KURT, IAN, DEL...

DEL?

DEL SHANNON, "RUNAWAY"?

125

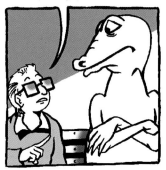

WHAT IS IT WITH THESE ANGST RIDDEN ARTIES WHO WANT TO RUN AWAY FROM THEMSELVES HEADLONG TO **EXTINCTION**?

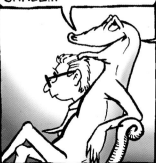

I THOUGHT **SHELLEY** PUT IT RATHER WELL, WHILE LYING 'BENEATH THE WILD WOOD'S GLOOMIEST SHADE...'

Would close my eyes and dream I were
On some remote and friendless plain,
And long to leave existence there,
If with it I might leave the pain
That with a cold finger and lean
Wrote madness on my withering mein.

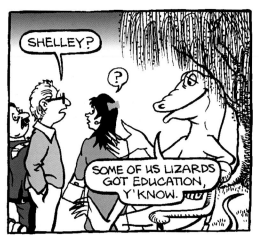

SHELLEY?

?

SOME OF US LIZARDS GOT EDUCATION, Y'KNOW.

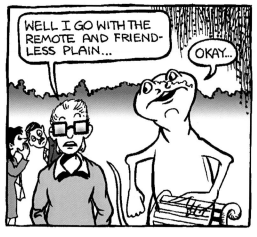

WELL I GO WITH THE REMOTE AND FRIENDLESS PLAIN...

OKAY...

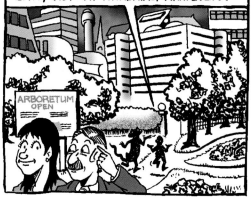

BUT MY URGE IS TO ESCAPE ALL **THIS** SHIT, NOT 'MY WITHERING WHATEVER'.

ARBORETUM
OPEN

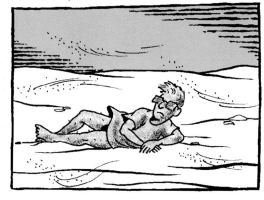

I LONG TO WAKE UP IN A VAST, HOSTILE **WILDERNESS**, ENVELOPED BY RAW NATURE, BLASTED BY THE ELEMENTS.

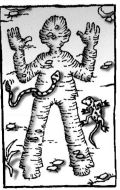

IT'S HOW I FEEL—EMPTY, BARREN, **DESOLATE**...

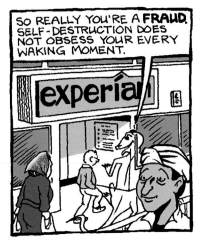

SO REALLY YOU'RE A **FRAUD**, SELF-DESTRUCTION DOES NOT OBSESS YOUR EVERY WAKING MOMENT.

experian

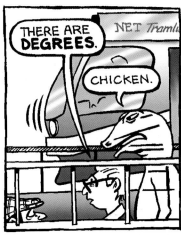

THERE ARE **DEGREES**.

CHICKEN.

NET Tramlu

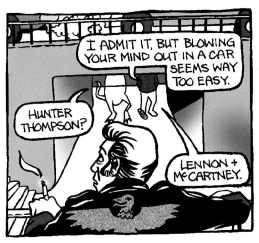

I ADMIT IT, BUT BLOWING YOUR MIND OUT IN A CAR SEEMS WAY TOO EASY.

HUNTER THOMPSON?

LENNON + McCARTNEY.

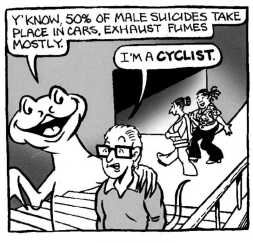

Y'KNOW, 50% OF MALE SUICIDES TAKE PLACE IN CARS, EXHAUST FUMES MOSTLY.

I'M A **CYCLIST**.

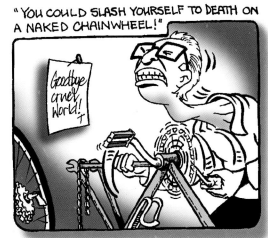

" YOU COULD SLASH YOURSELF TO DEATH ON A NAKED CHAINWHEEL!"

Goodbye cruel world! †

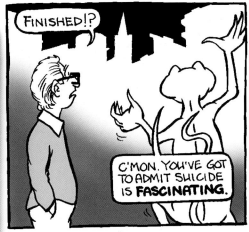

FINISHED!?

C'MON, YOU'VE GOT TO ADMIT SUICIDE IS **FASCINATING**.

127

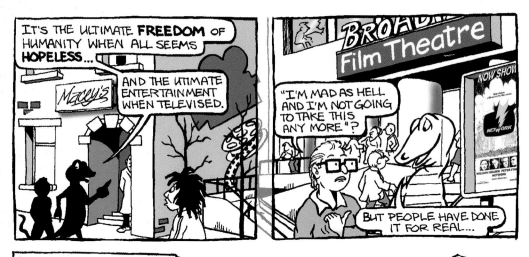

IT'S THE ULTIMATE **FREEDOM** OF HUMANITY WHEN ALL SEEMS **HOPELESS**...

AND THE ULTIMATE ENTERTAINMENT WHEN TELEVISED.

Macey's

BROAD Film Theatre

NOW SHOW

"I'M MAD AS HELL AND I'M NOT GOING TO TAKE THIS ANY MORE"?

NETWORK

BUT PEOPLE HAVE DONE IT FOR REAL...

"SHOT THEMSELVES ON T.V."

TV NEWSCASTER CHRISTINE CHUBBICK CRAVED A CLOSE RELATIONSHIP BUT WAS PLAGUED WITH LOW SELF-ESTEEM, DEPRESSION AND PERSISTENT ILLNESS. SHE WORKED FOR WXLT-TV IN FLORIDA, A STATION THAT LIKED TO PLAY UP 'BLOOD AND GUTS' STORIES, AND HAD BEEN RESEARCHING A PIECE ON SUICIDE THAT INCLUDED A LOCAL POLICE OFFICER'S TAKE ON THE MOST EFFECTIVE WAY TO SHOOT ONESELF. CHUBBICK'S LAST NEWSCAST INCLUDED A STORY ABOUT A RESTAURANT SHOOTING, BUT THE NEWSREEL JAMMED. ON SCREEN, SHE APOLOGISED FOR THE GLITCH AND SAID, 'IN KEEPING WITH CHANNEL 40'S POLICY OF BRINGING YOU THE LATEST IN BLOOD AND GUTS, AND IN LIVING COLOUR, YOU ARE GOING TO SEE ANOTHER FIRST.' SHE THEN PULLED OUT A 35 REVOLVER AND BLEW THE BACK OF HER HEAD OFF WITH A WADCUTTER TARGET BULLET, JUST AS THE COP RECOMMENDED.

CHARGED WITH RECEIVING A $300,000 KICKBACK WHILE STATE TREASURER, FORMER PENNSYLVANNIAN SENATOR BUDD DWYER PROFESSED TOTAL INNOCENCE AND REFUSED TO PLEA BARGAIN. FOUND GUILTY AND FACING A POSSIBLE 55 YEARS IN JAIL, DWYER CALLED A PRESS CONFERENCE THE DAY BEFORE SENTENCING TO EXPLAIN WHY AND HOW HE HAD BEEN MADE A POLITICAL SCAPEGOAT. AT THE CONFERENCE, HE HANDED THREE ENVELOPES TO HIS STAFF, LATER FOUND TO CONTAIN A SUICIDE NOTE TO HIS WIFE, HIS ORGAN DONOR CARD AND A LETTER TO THE NEW STATE GOVERNOR. FROM A FOURTH HE PULLED OUT A .357 MAGNUM AND SAID, 'PLEASE LEAVE THE ROOM IF THIS WILL OFFEND YOU.' THEN HE BLEW HIS BRAINS OUT IN FRONT OF FIVE LIVE TV CAMERAS.

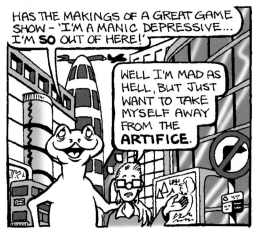

HAS THE MAKINGS OF A GREAT GAME SHOW – 'I'M A MANIC DEPRESSIVE... I'M **SO** OUT OF HERE!'

WELL I'M MAD AS HELL, BUT JUST WANT TO TAKE MYSELF AWAY FROM THE **ARTIFICE**.

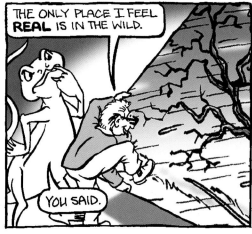

THE ONLY PLACE I FEEL **REAL** IS IN THE WILD.

YOU SAID.

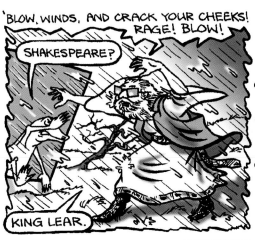

'BLOW, WINDS, AND CRACK YOUR CHEEKS! RAGE! BLOW!

SHAKESPEARE?

KING LEAR.

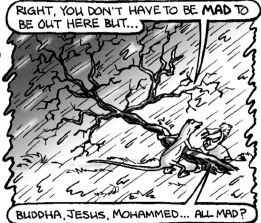

RIGHT, YOU DON'T HAVE TO BE **MAD** TO BE OUT HERE BUT...

BUDDHA, JESUS, MOHAMMED... ALL MAD?

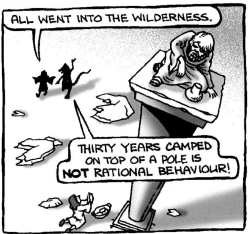

ALL WENT INTO THE WILDERNESS.

THIRTY YEARS CAMPED ON TOP OF A POLE IS **NOT** RATIONAL BEHAVIOUR!

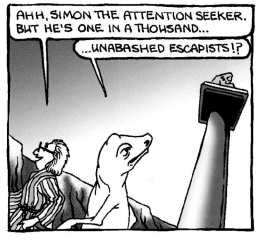

AHH, SIMON THE ATTENTION SEEKER. BUT HE'S ONE IN A THOUSAND...

...UNABASHED ESCAPISTS!?

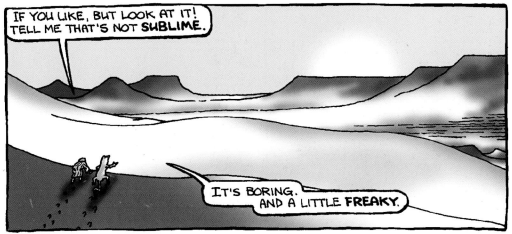

IF YOU LIKE, BUT LOOK AT IT! TELL ME THAT'S NOT **SUBLIME**.

IT'S BORING. AND A LITTLE **FREAKY**.

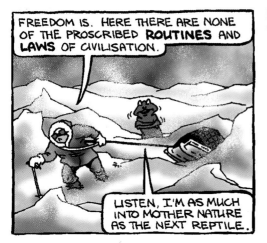

FREEDOM IS. HERE THERE ARE NONE OF THE PROSCRIBED **ROUTINES** AND **LAWS** OF CIVILISATION.

LISTEN, I'M AS MUCH INTO MOTHER NATURE AS THE NEXT REPTILE.

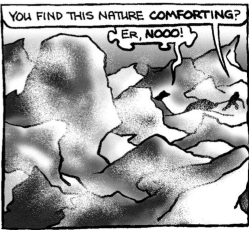

YOU FIND THIS NATURE **COMFORTING?**

ER, **NOOO!**

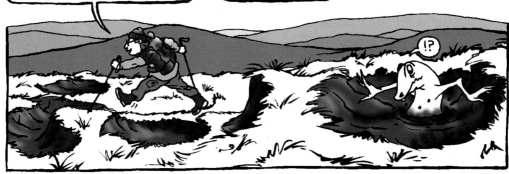

IT'S ALIEN, RAW, AUSTERE. DESERTS DON'T SUCKLE HUMAN BEINGS, BUT THEY CAN **LIBERATE** THEM... US.

THE PROPHETS CHOSE THE LANDSCAPE OF REVELATION OVER THE SOCIETY OF **SUFFOCATION.**

!?

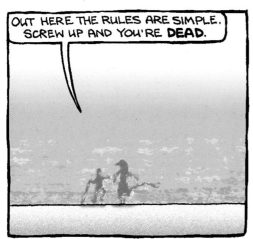

OUT HERE THE RULES ARE SIMPLE. SCREW UP AND YOU'RE **DEAD**.

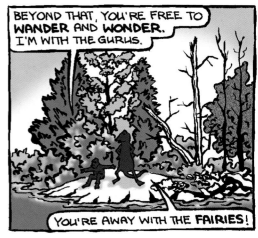

BEYOND THAT, YOU'RE FREE TO **WANDER** AND **WONDER**. I'M WITH THE GURUS.

YOU'RE AWAY WITH THE **FAIRIES!**

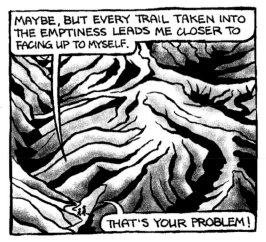

MAYBE, BUT EVERY TRAIL TAKEN INTO THE EMPTINESS LEADS ME CLOSER TO FACING UP TO MYSELF.

THAT'S YOUR PROBLEM!

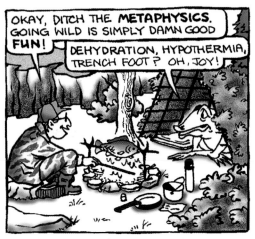

OKAY, DITCH THE **METAPHYSICS**. GOING WILD IS SIMPLY DAMN GOOD **FUN!**

DEHYDRATION, HYPOTHERMIA, TRENCH FOOT? OH, JOY!

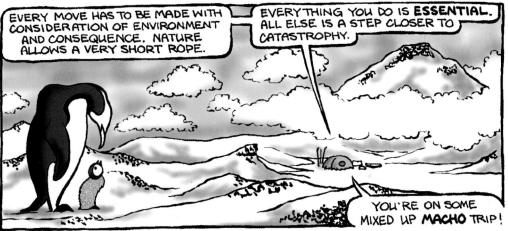

EVERY MOVE HAS TO BE MADE WITH CONSIDERATION OF ENVIRONMENT AND CONSEQUENCE. NATURE ALLOWS A VERY SHORT ROPE.

EVERYTHING YOU DO IS **ESSENTIAL**. ALL ELSE IS A STEP CLOSER TO CATASTROPHY.

YOU'RE ON SOME MIXED UP **MACHO** TRIP!

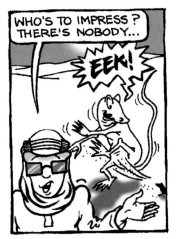

WHO'S TO IMPRESS? THERE'S NOBODY...

EEK!

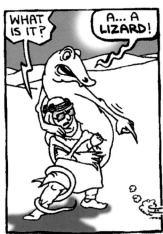

WHAT IS IT?

A... A LIZARD!

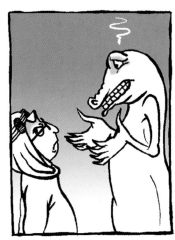

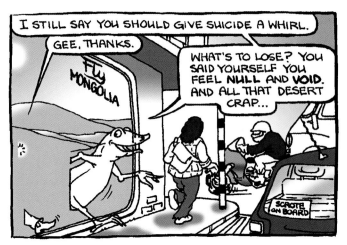

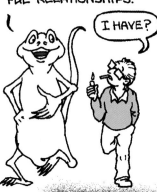

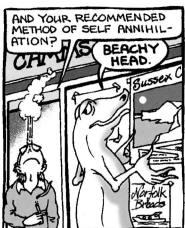

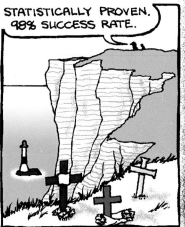

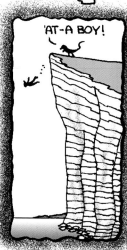

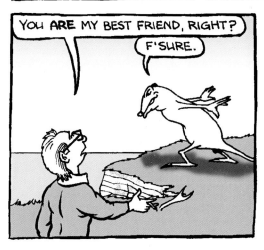

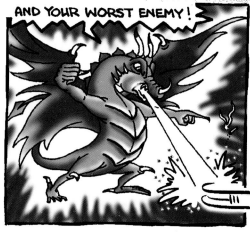

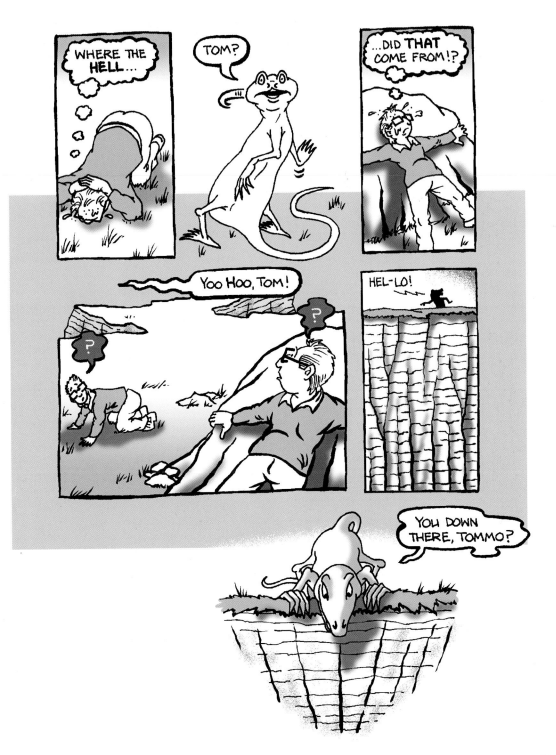

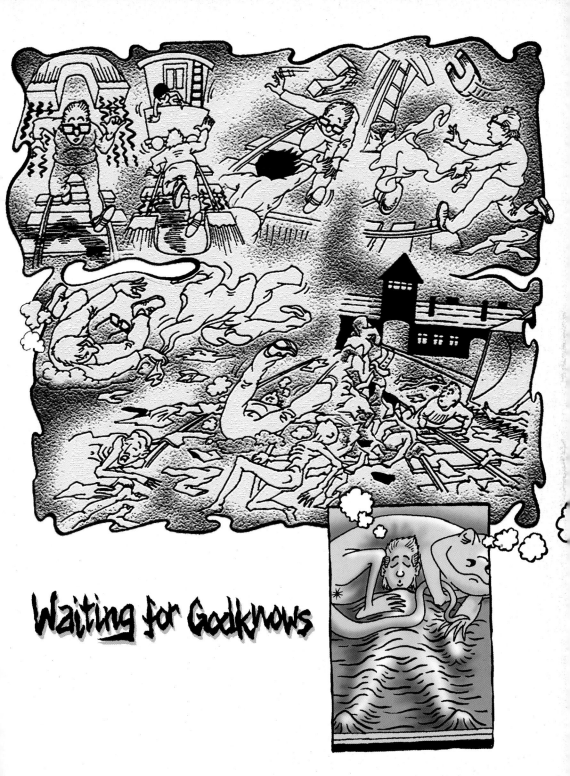

Waiting for Godknows

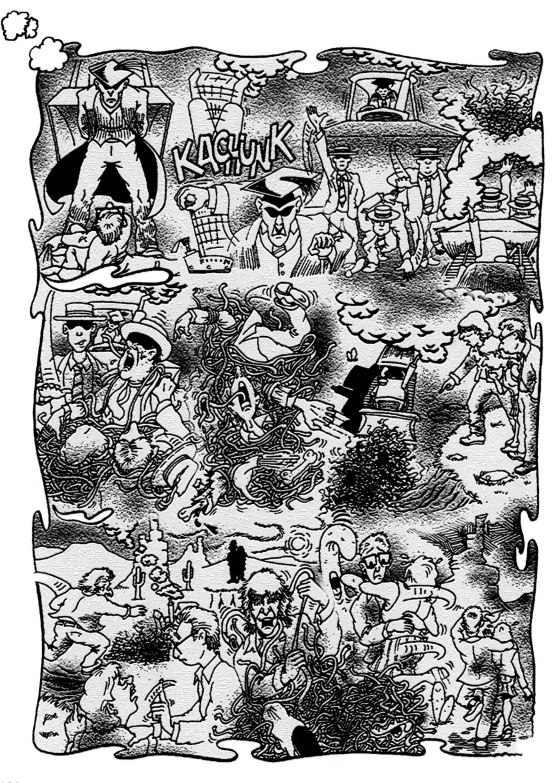

KACLUNK

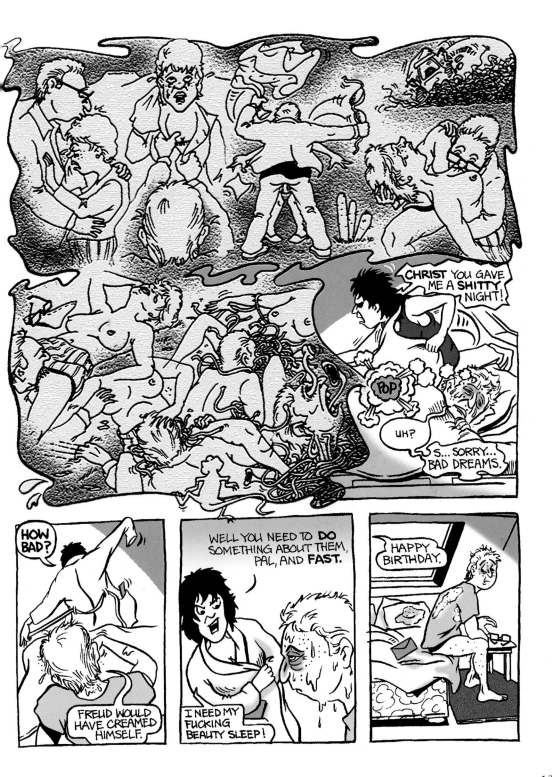

137

WHEREVER POSSIBLE, IT IS A **GOOD IDEA** TO PLAN FITS OF DEPRESSION SO THEY **DON'T** COINCIDE WITH YOUR BIRTHDAY.

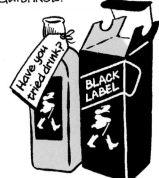

IF THAT'S A PROBLEM, **PLAN B** IS TO CASUALLY FOREWARN FRIENDS AND FAMILY THAT YOU ARE STRUGGLING TO FIND THE FUNNY SIDE OF **HIGH ANXIETY.**

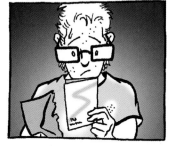

I FAILED ON BOTH COUNTS.

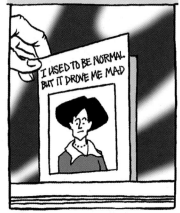

I USED TO BE NORMAL. BUT IT DROVE ME MAD

THUS I RECEIVED A BUNCH OF RIB-TICKLING PRESENTS ON MY DAY OF RECKONING...

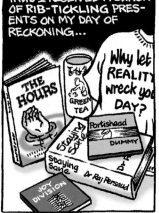

THE HOURS

Why let REALITY wreck you DAY?

GREEN TEA

Portishead
DUMMY

Staying Sane

staying sane Dr Raj Persaud

JOY DIVISION

AND A BOTTLE OF SCOTCH FROM MY DAD WITH A NOTE OF PARENTAL GUIDANCE.

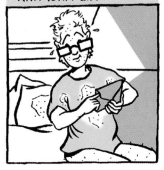

Have you tried drink?

BLACK LABEL

I ALSO FAILED TO PREDICT THAT JUDY WOULD ATTEMPT THE IMPOSSIBLE (TO CHEER ME UP) WITH THE IMPRUDENT (SHE THREW A PARTY).

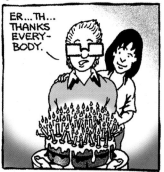

ER...TH... THANKS EVERY- BODY.

YOU'RE A COUPLE OF CANDLES SHORT OF THE FULL CAKE, BUT...

I...I DON'T KNOW WHAT TO SAY.

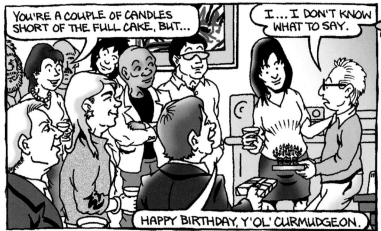

HAPPY BIRTHDAY, Y'OL' CURMUDGEON.

HOW ABOUT, "NOW BOG OFF AND LET ME GET BACK TO BEING MISER- ABLE IN PEACE"?

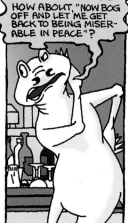

I ALWAYS FOUND OUR FRIENDS A LITTLE INTIMIDATING. IN A PACK THEY WERE **TERRIFYING.**

NOT WORTHY NOT WORTHY...

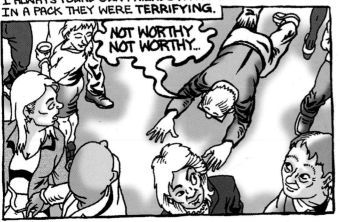

NEVER FIGURED OUT WHY THEY LIKE ME.

PROBABLY IT'S JUDY.

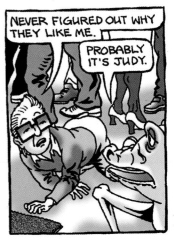

MUST BE. I MEAN, THEY'RE AT THE PEAK OF THEIR POWERS; CONFIDENT, SUCCESSFUL...

WELL-HEELED, GOING PLACES...

WHEREAS...

YOU'RE A FUCK-UP; LOUD-MOUTHED, ARROGANT...

BROKE, BUSTED...

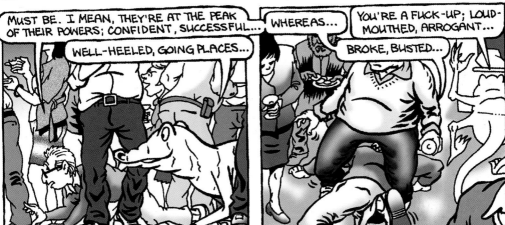

EXCEPT YOU CAN DRAW FUNNY PICTURES.

OH, WOW...

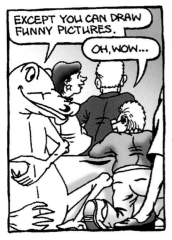

HOW OFTEN HAVE PEOPLE SAID THEY WISHED THEY COULD DO WHAT YOU DO?

ER... SO?

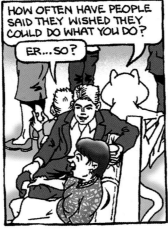

YOU THINK THEY SAY THAT TO BRAIN SURGEONS?

OKAY, BUT I... I CAN'T DO IT ANY MORE!

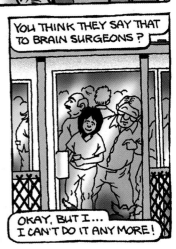

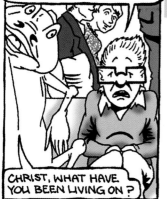

I HAVEN'T PUT PEN TO PAPER SINCE WE LEFT FOR CHINA.

CHRIST, WHAT HAVE YOU BEEN LIVING ON?

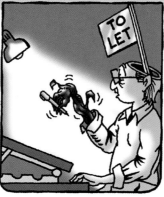

THE ONE SKILL THAT GAVE ME A SMIDGEN OF SELF-ESTEEM HAD WITHERED ON THE VINE.

TO LET

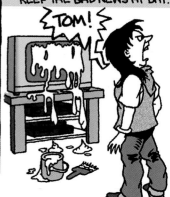

I HAD NO INTEREST IN WHAT WAS GOING ON IN THE WORLD AND MADE EVERY EFFORT TO KEEP THE BAD NEWS AT BAY.

TOM!

THE FACES MIGHT HAVE CHANGED, BUT SURE AS THE POPE'S A FUNDAMENTALIST THE SAME OLD HORSEMEN WERE STILL RIDING POINT FOR THE SAME OLD LUNATIC PURPOSES.

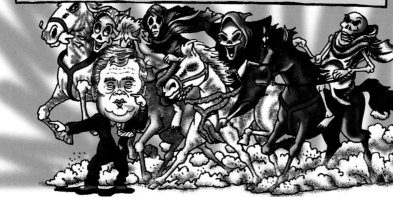

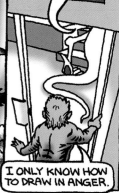

SO DRAW SOMETHING **NICE** FOR A CHANGE.

I ONLY KNOW HOW TO DRAW IN ANGER.

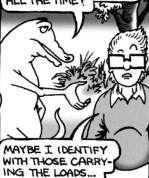

F'CHRISSAKE, WHY THE NEED TO TAKE ON THE BURDENS OF THE WORLD ALL THE TIME?

MAYBE I IDENTIFY WITH THOSE CARRYING THE LOADS...

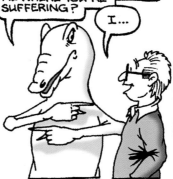

REALLY!? LOOK ABOUT YOU, TOM. NICE HOME, LOVELY MISSUS, GREAT JOB... TELL ME WHERE YOU'RE SUFFERING?

I...

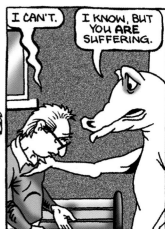

I CAN'T.

I KNOW, BUT YOU **ARE** SUFFERING.

140

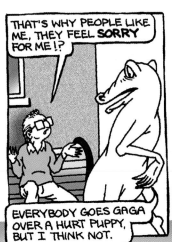

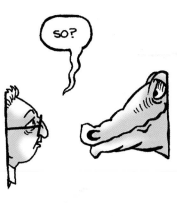

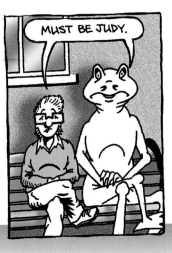

I WAS MISERABLE ALRIGHT, BUT LIFE WAS HARDLY PEACEFUL. ASIDE FROM THE PERSISTENT MONOLOGUE OF DELIBERATIONS ON DELIBERATIONS, THERE WAS THE POSTMAN OR MEN.

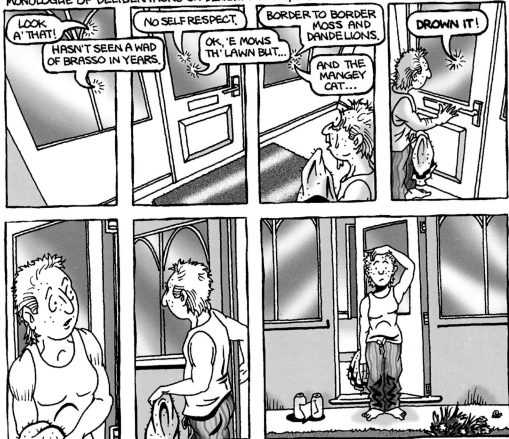

141

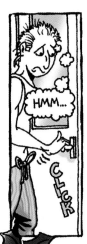

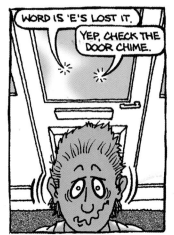

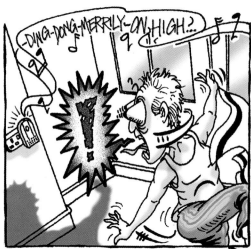

CHRISTMAS IS ANOTHER CELEBRATION BEST AVOIDED BY DEPRESSOS (HEAD FOR A MUSLIM COUNTRY WITHOUT PASSING THROUGH HEATHROW).

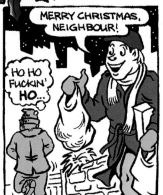

MY PROBLEM WITH THE SEASON OF RAPACIOUS CONSUMPTION WAS THE LEVEL OF ACCEPTABLE INSANITY.

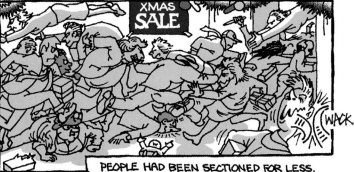

PEOPLE HAD BEEN SECTIONED FOR LESS.

BY CHRISTMAS EVE, I WAS THE ONLY SANE BUGGER ON THE BLOCK. HALF THE NATION WERE SUICIDAL, THE OTHER HALF HOMICIDAL.

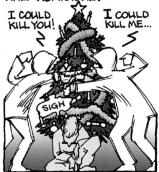

UTTER DESPAIR CAN BE AVOIDED, HOWEVER, BY INVITING TO THE TABLE SOMEONE EVEN MORE DELUDED THAN YOURSELF.

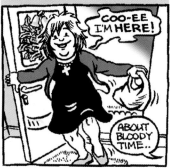

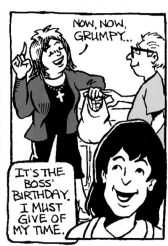

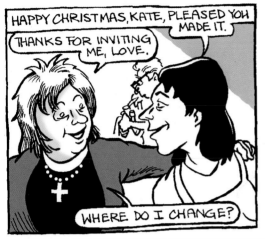

HAPPY CHRISTMAS, KATE, PLEASED YOU MADE IT.

THANKS FOR INVITING ME, LOVE.

WHERE DO I CHANGE?

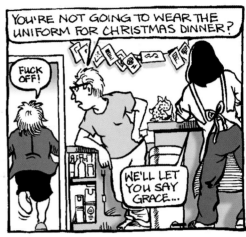

YOU'RE NOT GOING TO WEAR THE UNIFORM FOR CHRISTMAS DINNER?

FUCK OFF!

WE'LL LET YOU SAY GRACE...

FOR EIGHT YEARS JUDY AND MYSELF HAD TRIED TO DISSUADE OUR FRIEND FROM BECOMING A PRIEST.

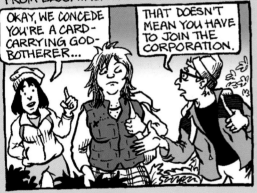

OKAY, WE CONCEDE YOU'RE A CARD-CARRYING GOD-BOTHERER...

THAT DOESN'T MEAN YOU HAVE TO JOIN THE CORPORATION.

KATE WAS A NURSE AND A GOOD ONE. WITH HER SKILLS, FAITH AND DOWN-TO-EARTH PERSONALITY SHE COULD HAVE HEALED WAR-TORN BODIES AND SOULS.

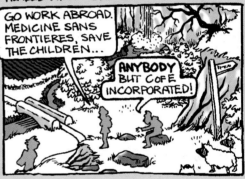

GO WORK ABROAD. MEDICINE SANS FRONTIERES, SAVE THE CHILDREN...

ANYBODY BUT CofE INCORPORATED!

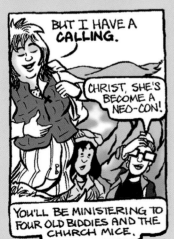

BUT I HAVE A CALLING.

CHRIST, SHE'S BECOME A NEO-CON!

YOU'LL BE MINISTERING TO FOUR OLD BIDDIES AND THE CHURCH MICE.

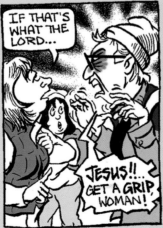

IF THAT'S WHAT THE LORD...

JESUS!!... GET A GRIP, WOMAN!

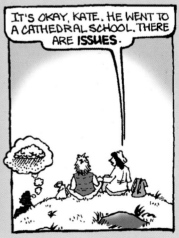

IT'S OKAY, KATE. HE WENT TO A CATHEDRAL SCHOOL. THERE ARE ISSUES.

143

KATE WAS BANGING ON THE CHURCH DOOR AND FIELDING HARD BALL FROM FRIENDS FOR ALMOST A DECADE. I FIGURED SHE HAD TO KNOW A THING OR TWO ABOUT **BELIEF**. SOMETHING I WAS BEGINNING TO WONDER ABOUT.

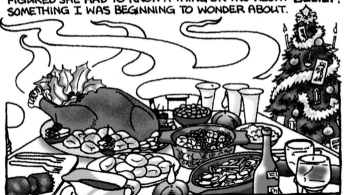

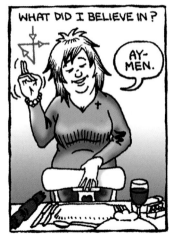

WHAT DID I BELIEVE IN?

AY-MEN.

CLEARLY NOT MYSELF, BUT DID ANY ASPECT OF THE HUMAN AGENDA IGNITE A FLICKER OF FAITH IN ME?

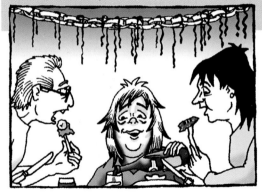

OR WAS I DOWN WITH TERMINAL JAUNDICE THE SOUL, DRAINED OF SPIRIT, PEGGED OUT AND YELLOWING IN AN EMOTIONAL WASTELAND?

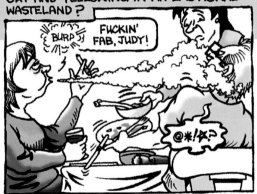

BURP

FUCKIN' FAB, JUDY!

@*!¥?

WAS I IN DIRE NEED OF SOME OF THAT OL' TIME RELIGION...?

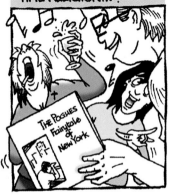

THE POGUES Fairytale of New York

INVITING KATE FOR DINNER, I HOPED TO STEAL A BLOATED MOMENT FOR A QUIET CHAT ABOUT MATTERS SPIRITUAL.

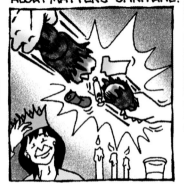

NOTHING TOO HEAVY FOR CHRISTMAS DAY...

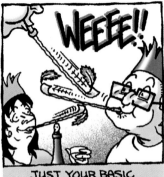

WEEEE!!

JUST YOUR BASIC EXISTENTIAL CONUNDRUMS.

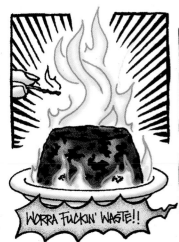

WORRA FUCKIN' WASTE!!

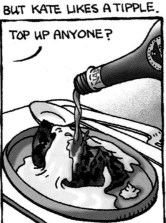

BUT KATE LIKES A TIPPLE.

TOP UP ANYONE?

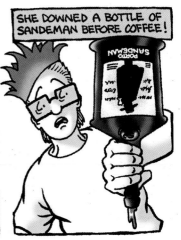

SHE DOWNED A BOTTLE OF SANDEMAN BEFORE COFFEE!

SO THE BLOATED MOMENT BECAME MENTAL ROUNDS OF MUSICAL CHAIRS...

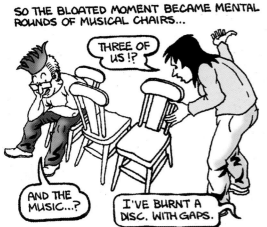

THREE OF US!?

AND THE MUSIC...?

I'VE BURNT A DISC. WITH GAPS.

AND INTERMINABLE CHARADES.

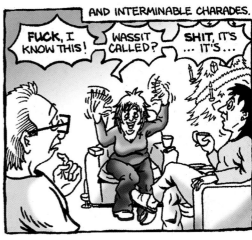

FUCK, I KNOW THIS!

WASSIT CALLED?

SHIT, IT'S ... IT'S ...

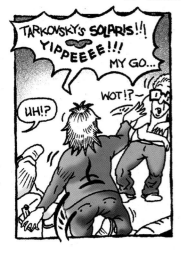

TARKOVSKY'S SOLARIS!!!
YIPPEEEE!!!
MY GO...

UH!?

WOT!?—

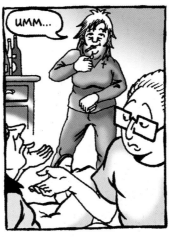

UMM...

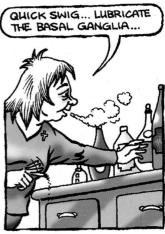

QUICK SWIG... LUBRICATE THE BASAL GANGLIA...

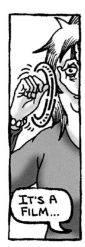 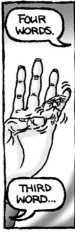 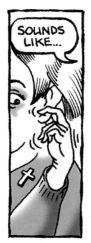 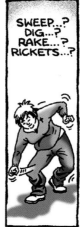 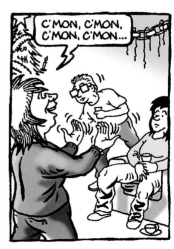

FOUR WORDS.

IT'S A FILM...

THIRD WORD...

SOUNDS LIKE...

SWEEP...? DIG...? RAKE...? RICKETS...?

C'MON, C'MON, C'MON, C'MON...

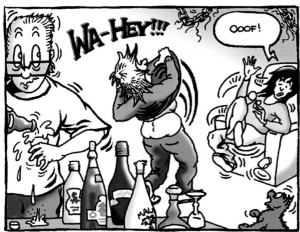 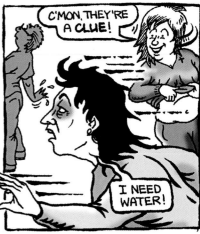

WA-HEY!!!

OOOF!

C'MON, THEY'RE A CLUE!

I NEED WATER!

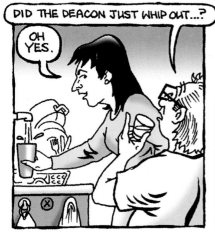 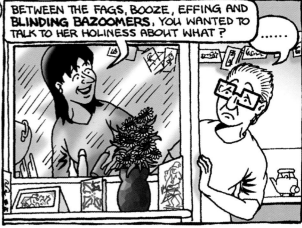

DID THE DEACON JUST WHIP OUT...?

OH YES.

BETWEEN THE FAGS, BOOZE, EFFING AND **BLINDING BAZOOMERS**, YOU WANTED TO TALK TO HER HOLINESS ABOUT WHAT?

......

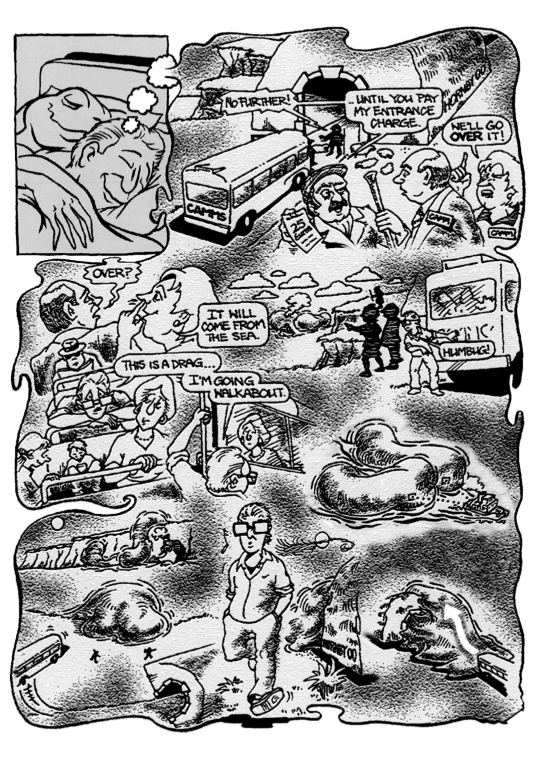

147

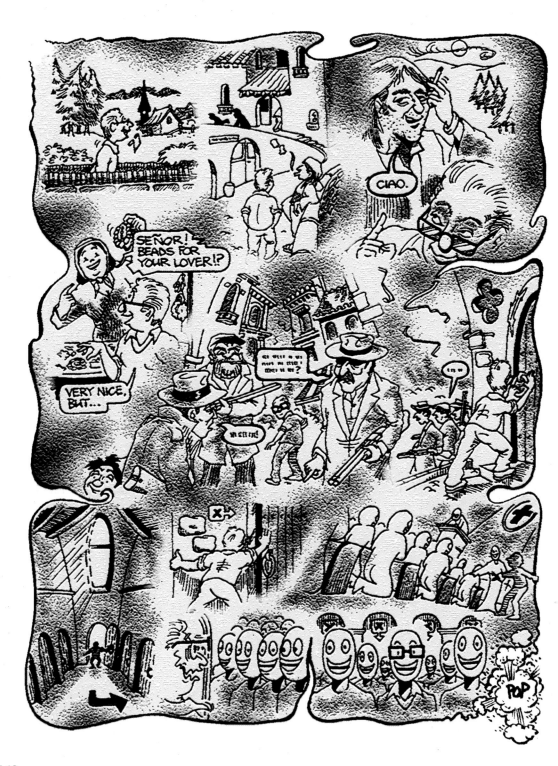

148

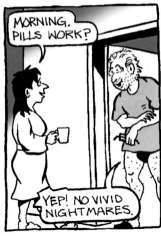

MORNING. PILLS WORK?

YEP! NO VIVID NIGHTMARES.

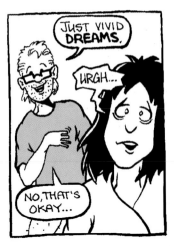

JUST VIVID DREAMS.

URGH...

NO, THAT'S OKAY...

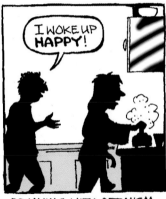

I WOKE UP HAPPY!

BRIMMING WITH OPTIMISM, RARING TO GO, HUNGRY FOR THE MIGHTY DOLLAR?

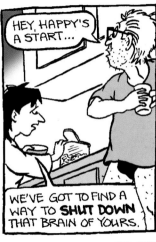

HEY, HAPPY'S A START...

WE'VE GOT TO FIND A WAY TO **SHUT DOWN** THAT BRAIN OF YOURS.

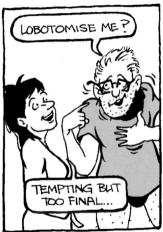

LOBOTOMISE ME?

TEMPTING BUT TOO FINAL....

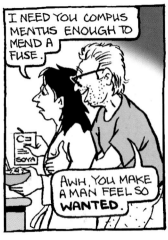

I NEED YOU COMPUS MENTUS ENOUGH TO MEND A FUSE.

SOYA

AWH, YOU MAKE A MAN FEEL SO **WANTED**.

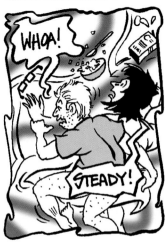

WHOA!

STEADY!

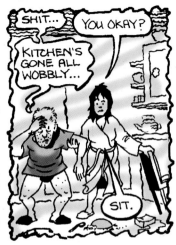

SHIT...

YOU OKAY?

KITCHEN'S GONE ALL WOBBLY...

SIT.

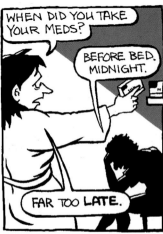

WHEN DID YOU TAKE YOUR MEDS?

BEFORE BED, MIDNIGHT.

FAR TOO **LATE**.

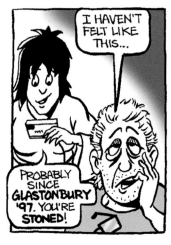

I HAVEN'T FELT LIKE THIS...

PROBABLY SINCE **GLASTONBURY** '97. YOU'RE **STONED!**

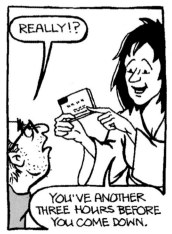

REALLY!?

YOU'VE ANOTHER THREE HOURS BEFORE YOU COME DOWN.

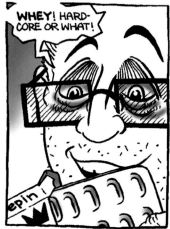

WHEY! HARD-CORE OR WHAT!

40mg OF CITALOPRAM HAD BEEN REPLACED BY 75mg OF **DOSULEPIN HYDROCHLORIDE,** USED "TO TREAT DEPRESSION, ESPECIALLY WHERE AN ANTI-ANXIETY EFFECT IS REQUIRED," THE LEAFLET SAID. ACCORDING TO DR. TWITCH...

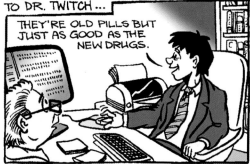

THEY'RE OLD PILLS BUT JUST AS GOOD AS THE NEW DRUGS.

THIS SORT OF CONTRADICTED WHAT HE SAID WHEN I **FIRST** WENT TO SEE HIM.

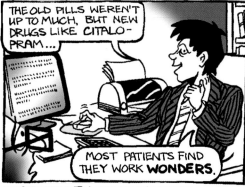

THE OLD PILLS WEREN'T UP TO MUCH, BUT NEW DRUGS LIKE CITALO-PRAM...

MOST PATIENTS FIND THEY WORK **WONDERS.**

EVIDENTLY I WASN'T 'MOST PATIENTS'...

MY NEW OLD PILLS TOOK ABOUT **TWO HOURS** TO KNOCK ME OUT, DURING WHICH TIME MY BRAIN WENT **BERSERK.**

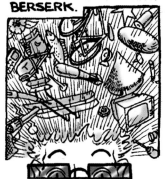

I SLEPT FOR ENGLAND AND GENERALLY DIDN'T DREAM. IF I DID, IT WAS IN SHORT BURSTS AND SURROUND SOUND, RICH IN TOUCH, TASTE AND SMELLS.

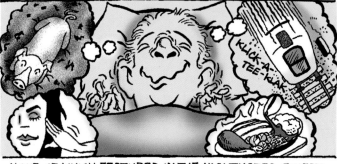

KLICK-A-TEE-KLAK

NONE OF WHICH FEATURED IN THE NIGHTMARES, EXCEPT FOR THE ODD STARTLING SOUND EFFECT FOR ADDED TERROR.

150

WHEN I AWOKE IT WAS AS FROM A HEAVY ANAES-THETIC; LIKE TRYING TO CRAWL UP LOOSE SAND.

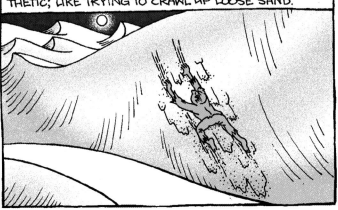

"DOSULEPIN CAN MAKE YOU DROWSY," THE LEAFLET WARNED, "DO NOT OPERATE MACHINERY OR DO ANYTHING THAT REQUIRES YOU TO BE **ALERT**"... WHICH REALLY CRAMPED MY **MODUS VIVENDI**.

CYCLING BECAME A PROBLEM...

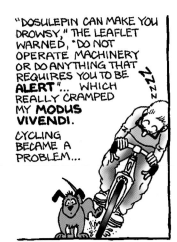

WALKING WASN'T MUCH EASIER.

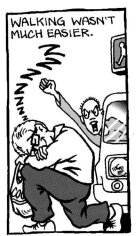

DRAWING...

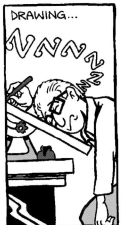

READING...

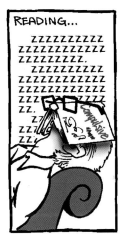

... EVEN THINKING BECAME A MAJOR CHALLENGE.

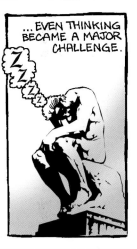

ABOUT THE ONLY ASPECT OF MY LIFE THAT DOSULEPIN IMPROVED WAS MY CONDUCT BEHIND THE WHEEL. SUDDENLY I WAS THE KNIGHT ROYAL OF THE ROAD.

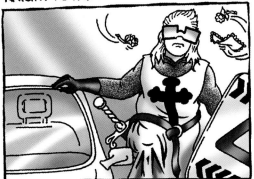

TUFTY FLUFFYTAIL COULD NOT HAVE BEEN MORE ACCOMMODATING OF VULNERABLE USERS. I GOT FAN MAIL FROM LOLLIPOP LADIES.

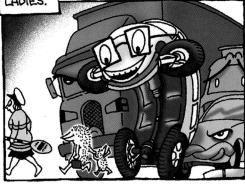

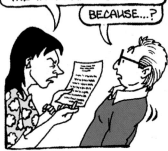

THEN IT WAS EXPLAINED THAT 'DO NOT OPERATE MACHINERY' = DRIVING.

IF YOU MUST USE THE CAR, WE'VE GOT TO INFORM THE INSURANCE COMPANY.

BECAUSE...?

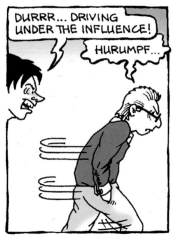

DURRR... DRIVING UNDER THE INFLUENCE!

HURUMPF...

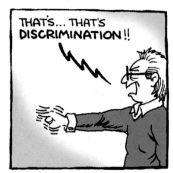

THAT'S... THAT'S **DISCRIMINATION**!!

JUDY WAS RIGHT. I WAS A CLEAR AND PRESENT DANGER. I ABJECTLY FAILED TO FOLLOW ALL KINDS OF STANDARD DRIVING PRACTICES.

I FORGOT TO...

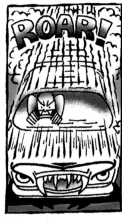

ROAR!

NEGLECTED TO...

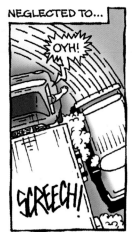

OYH!

SCREECH!

FAILED TO...

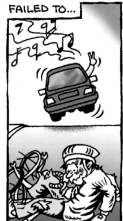

AND NEVER...

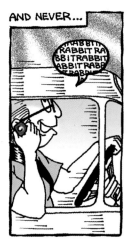

RABBIT RABBIT RABBIT RABBIT RABBIT RABBIT RABBIT RABBIT

SEEMED THE ONLY THING I WAS FIT FOR WAS VEGGING OUT ON '**THE X FACTOR**'.

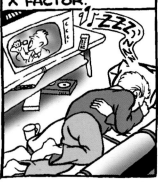

ZZZ

THE WORLD ABOUT ME WAS DEGENERATING INTO A MESS OF **SLURRY**, BUT I PERSEVERED WITH THE MEDS.

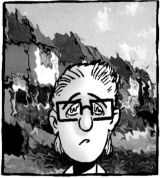

AND SO I WAITED FOR THE DAY DOSULEPIN **CURED** ME.

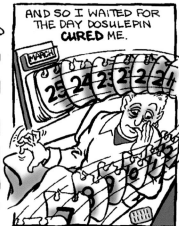

MARCH

I WAITED...

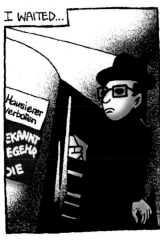

AND WAITED...

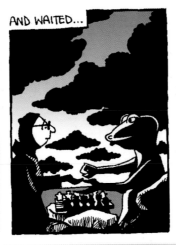

AND **WAITED.**

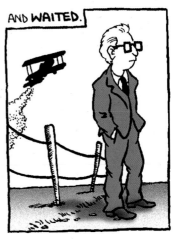

MEANTIME I WAS REFERRED TO THE **N**ATIONAL **C**OUNSELLING **S**ERVICE AND SENT A PROBING QUESTIONAIRE.

SHIT, IF I KNEW THE ANSWERS TO THIS LOT I WOULDN'T FUCKIN' NEED COUNSELLING!

LANGUAGE!

THREE MONTHS LATER I RECEIVED AN APPOINT- MENT. THEIR OFFICE WASN'T EASY TO FIND.

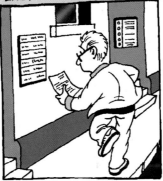

IT WAS EVEN HARDER TO FIND WITHOUT BEING **NOTICED!**

HEY, TOM, WHATCHA DOIN' THIS SIDE OF TOWN?

I, ER... THAT IS...

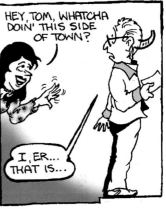

AT RECEPTION I HAD TO FILL IN **ANOTHER** QUESTIONAIRE.

LET ME GUESS... YOU WANT TO KNOW IF I'VE COMMITTED SUICIDE LATELY.

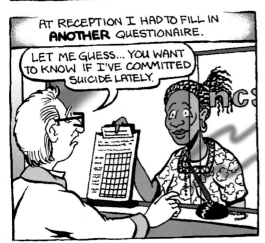

FINALLY I GOT TO MEET MARTINE, A SENIOR COUNSELLOR. SHE WAS INFORMAL, PLEASANT AND **OBESE.**

YOU NEED COUNSELLING, MY GIRL...

JUST GOT A FEW QUESTIONS, TOM...

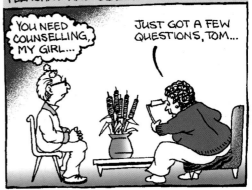

FOR AN HOUR MARTINE 'INTERVIEWED' ME, BUT I LEARNED A FEW THINGS ABOUT MYSELF ALONG THE WAY.

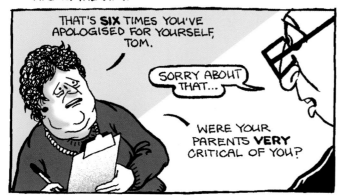

THAT'S **SIX** TIMES YOU'VE APOLOGISED FOR YOURSELF, TOM.

SORRY ABOUT THAT...

WERE YOUR PARENTS **VERY** CRITICAL OF YOU?

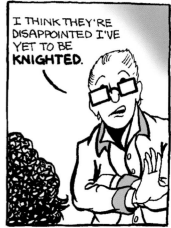

I THINK THEY'RE DISAPPOINTED I'VE YET TO BE **KNIGHTED.**

AND I LEARNED A FEW THINGS ABOUT THE MENTAL HEALTH PROFESSION.

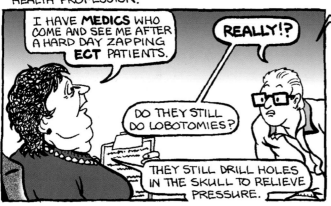

I HAVE **MEDICS** WHO COME AND SEE ME AFTER A HARD DAY ZAPPING **ECT** PATIENTS.

REALLY!?

DO THEY STILL DO LOBOTOMIES?

THEY STILL DRILL HOLES IN THE SKULL TO RELIEVE PRESSURE.

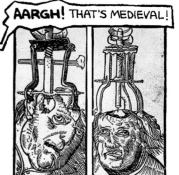

AARGH! THAT'S MEDIEVAL!

"PREHISTORIC, ACTUALLY, BUT IN THE U.S.A. THEY'RE QUEUEING UP FOR ELECTIVE **TREPANATION."**

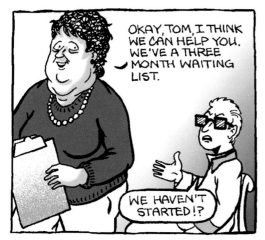

OKAY, TOM, I THINK WE CAN HELP YOU. WE'VE A THREE MONTH WAITING LIST.

WE HAVEN'T STARTED!?

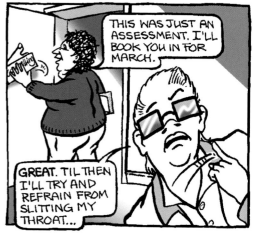

THIS WAS JUST AN ASSESSMENT. I'LL BOOK YOU IN FOR MARCH.

GREAT. TIL THEN I'LL TRY AND REFRAIN FROM SLITTING MY THROAT...

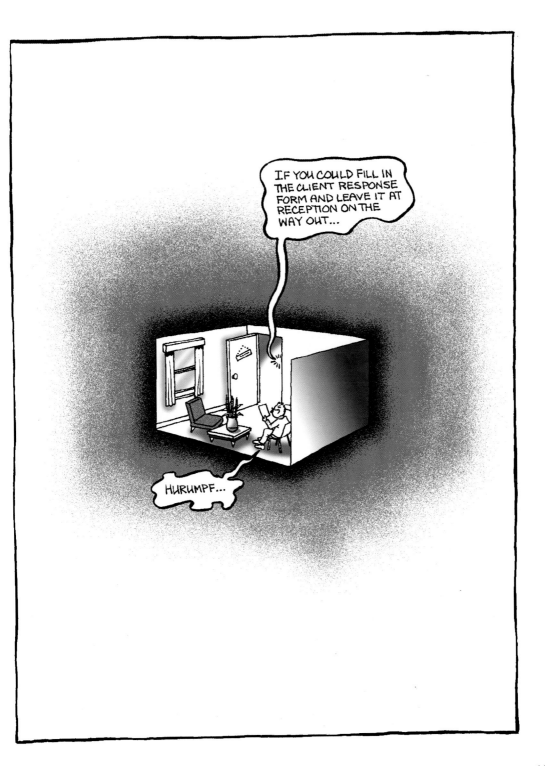

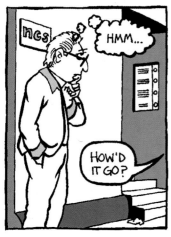

HMM...

HOW'D IT GO?

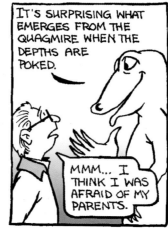

IT'S SURPRISING WHAT EMERGES FROM THE QUAGMIRE WHEN THE DEPTHS ARE POKED.

MMM... I THINK I WAS AFRAID OF MY PARENTS.

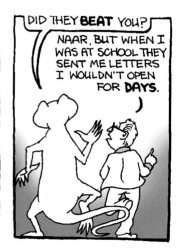

DID THEY **BEAT** YOU?

NAAR, BUT WHEN I WAS AT SCHOOL THEY SENT ME LETTERS I WOULDN'T OPEN FOR **DAYS**.

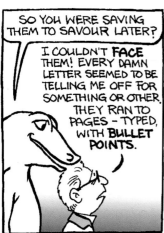

SO YOU WERE SAVING THEM TO SAVOUR LATER?

I COULDN'T **FACE** THEM! EVERY DAMN LETTER SEEMED TO BE TELLING ME OFF FOR SOMETHING OR OTHER. THEY RAN TO PAGES - TYPED, WITH **BULLET POINTS**.

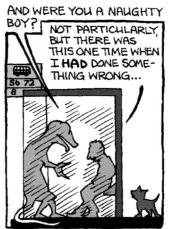

AND WERE YOU A NAUGHTY BOY?

NOT PARTICULARLY, BUT THERE WAS THIS ONE TIME WHEN I **HAD** DONE SOMETHING WRONG...

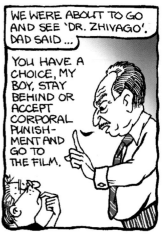

WE WERE ABOUT TO GO AND SEE 'DR. ZHIVAGO'. DAD SAID ...

YOU HAVE A CHOICE, MY BOY, STAY BEHIND OR ACCEPT CORPORAL PUNISHMENT AND GO TO THE FILM.

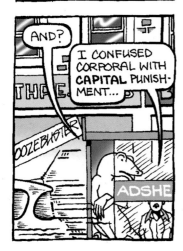

AND?

I CONFUSED CORPORAL WITH **CAPITAL** PUNISHMENT...

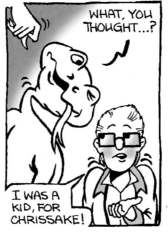

WHAT, YOU THOUGHT...?

I WAS A KID, FOR CHRISSAKE!

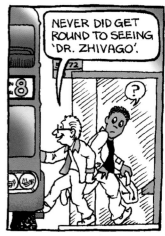

NEVER DID GET ROUND TO SEEING 'DR. ZHIVAGO'.

?

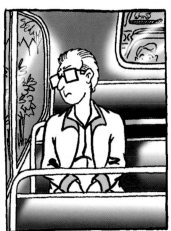

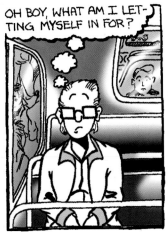
OH BOY, WHAT AM I LETTING MYSELF IN FOR?

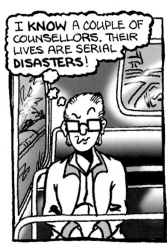
I KNOW A COUPLE OF COUNSELLORS. THEIR LIVES ARE SERIAL DISASTERS!

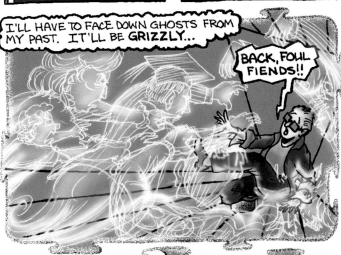
I'LL HAVE TO FACE DOWN GHOSTS FROM MY PAST. IT'LL BE GRIZZLY...

BACK, FOUL FIENDS!!

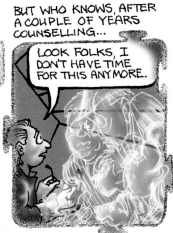
BUT WHO KNOWS, AFTER A COUPLE OF YEARS COUNSELLING...

LOOK FOLKS, I DON'T HAVE TIME FOR THIS ANYMORE.

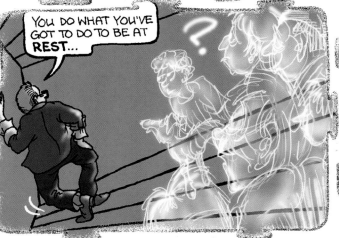
YOU DO WHAT YOU'VE GOT TO DO TO BE AT REST...

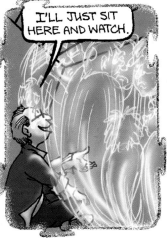
I'LL JUST SIT HERE AND WATCH.

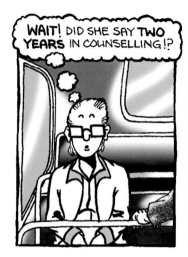

WAIT! DID SHE SAY **TWO YEARS** IN COUNSELLING!?

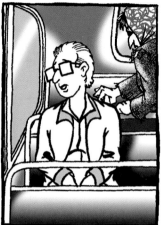

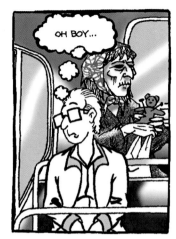

OH BOY...

SO I CONTINUED WITH THE **MEDS** AND WENT BACK TO WAITING...

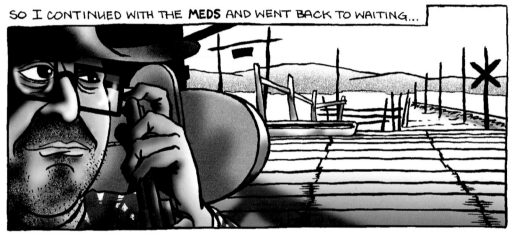

AND WAITING...

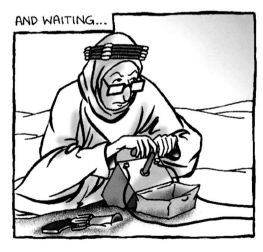

AND **WAITING.**

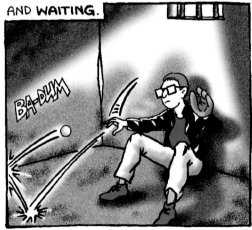

BA-DUM

IF YOU HAVEN'T THE DOSH TO GO **PRIVATE**, YOU NEED THE PATIENCE OF A CICADA WAITING FOR THE HEALTH SERVICE TO GET ROUND TO YOU.

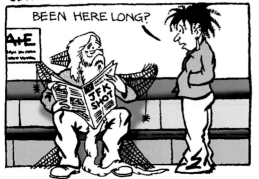

BEEN HERE LONG?

17 YEARS CICADAS LIVE UNDERGROUND BEFORE THEY BREAK OUT, COLONISE A TREE AND SHAG THEMSELVES STUPID.

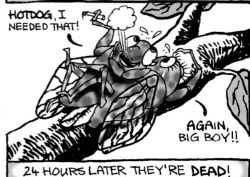

HOTDOG, I NEEDED THAT!

AGAIN, BIG BOY!!

24 HOURS LATER THEY'RE **DEAD**!

COINCIDENTALLY, 17 WEEKS AFTER I STARTED ON DOSULEPIN, A HAREM OF CICADAS COLONISED MY **SKULL**.

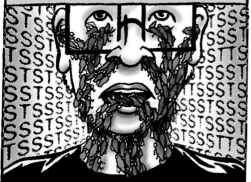

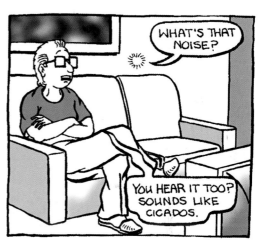

WHAT'S THAT NOISE?

YOU HEAR IT TOO? SOUNDS LIKE CICADOS.

RIGHT. CERTANLY NOT CRICKETS.

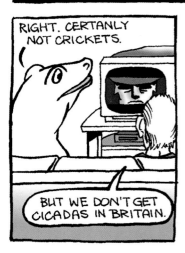

BUT WE DON'T GET CICADAS IN BRITAIN.

RIGHT AGAIN.

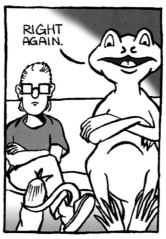

OH, SHIT.

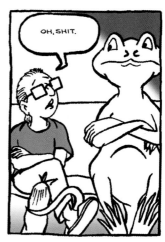

IT SOUNDS NOTHING LIKE BELLS, BUT IT IS DESCRIBED AS RINGING IN THE EARS, AKA **TINNITUS.**

HOW SOON BEFORE BATTLES START RAGING?

OR WORSE.

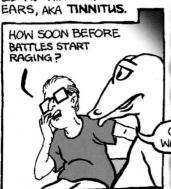

DINNER'S UP, DEAR!

I'LL TAKE IT IN MY TENT...

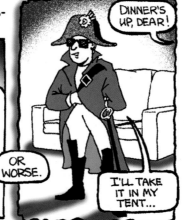

SO IT WAS BACK DOWN THE DOC'S TO CHANGE THE MEDS.

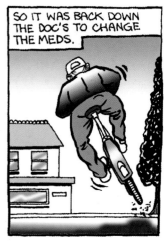

'... ENLARGED BREASTS, OVER-PRODUCTION OF BREAST MILK...'

I'M EXPRESSING IT FOR THE THIRD WORLD.

'... TREMOR, DIZZINESS, **TINNITUS.'** RIGHT, IT **IS** A SIDE EFFECT OF 'DOSULEPIN.'

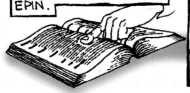

OKAY, LET'S TRY YOU ON **AMITRIPTYLINE.**

HELL, WHY NOT.

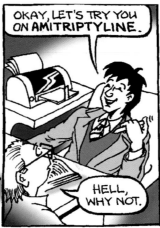

WE NEED TO FIND SOMETHING THAT **CHILLS** YOU WITHOUT ZOMBIFYING THE LIFE OUT OF YOU.

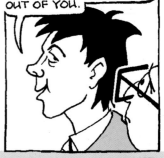

THIS WAS BECOMING TREATMENT BY SUCK-IT-AND-SEE!

A YEAR ON FROM STARTING THE MEDS I HAD PUMPED INTO MY SYSTEM LARGE QUANTITIES OF...

• CITALOPRAM HYDROBROMIDE
• DOSULEPIN HYDROCHLORIDE
• AMITRIPTYLINE HYDROCHLORIDE • MAGNESIUM STEARATE
• COLLOIDAL ANHYDROUS SILICA

(NOT TO MENTION THE RAFT OF 'E' NUMBERS THAT CONSTITUTE TABLET COATINGS AND CAPSULE SHELLS).

TO A LAYMAN LIKE ME THAT SOUNDED A **HEADY** COCKTAIL OF CHEMICALS.

MOSTLY BENIGN, THEY WERE ALSO 'POTENTIALLY **LIFE-THREATENING',** ACCORDING TO THE BLURB.
I MENTIONED MY IN-TAKE TO NURSE-CUM-VICAR, KATE. HER COMMENT...

HMM... -INES, -INS, -IDES...

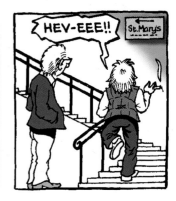

HEV-EEE!!

St.Marys

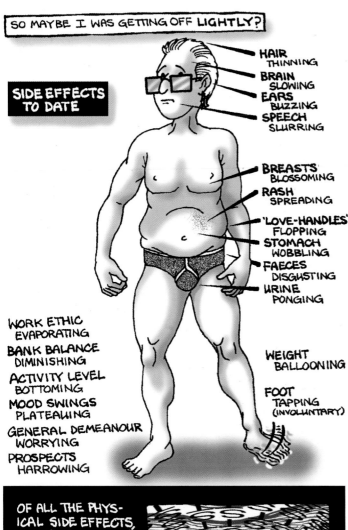

SO MAYBE I WAS GETTING OFF **LIGHTLY?**

SIDE EFFECTS TO DATE

HAIR
THINNING

BRAIN
SLOWING

EARS
BUZZING

SPEECH
SLURRING

BREASTS
BLOSSOMING

RASH
SPREADING

'LOVE-HANDLES'
FLOPPING

STOMACH
WOBBLING

FAECES
DISGUSTING

URINE
PONGING

WORK ETHIC
EVAPORATING

BANK BALANCE
DIMINISHING

ACTIVITY LEVEL
BOTTOMING

MOOD SWINGS
PLATEAUING

GENERAL DEMEANOUR
WORRYING

PROSPECTS
HARROWING

WEIGHT
BALLOONING

FOOT
TAPPING
(INVOLUNTARY)

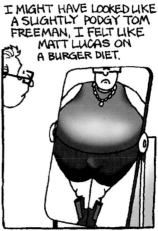

I MIGHT HAVE LOOKED LIKE A SLIGHTLY PODGY TOM FREEMAN, I FELT LIKE MATT LUCAS ON A BURGER DIET.

AND FOR WHAT!?

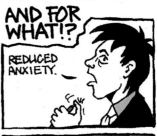

REDUCED ANXIETY.

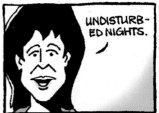

UNDISTURB-ED NIGHTS.

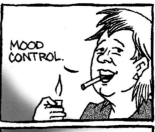

MOOD CONTROL.

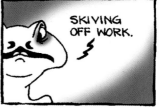

SKIVING OFF WORK.

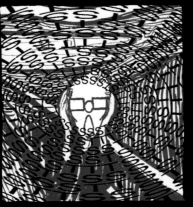

OF ALL THE PHYSICAL SIDE EFFECTS, TINNITUS WAS THE MOST INTOLERABLE. WHITE NOISE SCREAMING IN YOUR EARS 24-7 IS NOTHING SHORT OF TORTUROUS.

ON THE UPSIDE, THERE WERE DAYS WHEN THE HISSSS WAS THE ONLY CONFIRMATION THAT I HAD NOT JOINED THE RANKS OF THE UNDEAD!

161

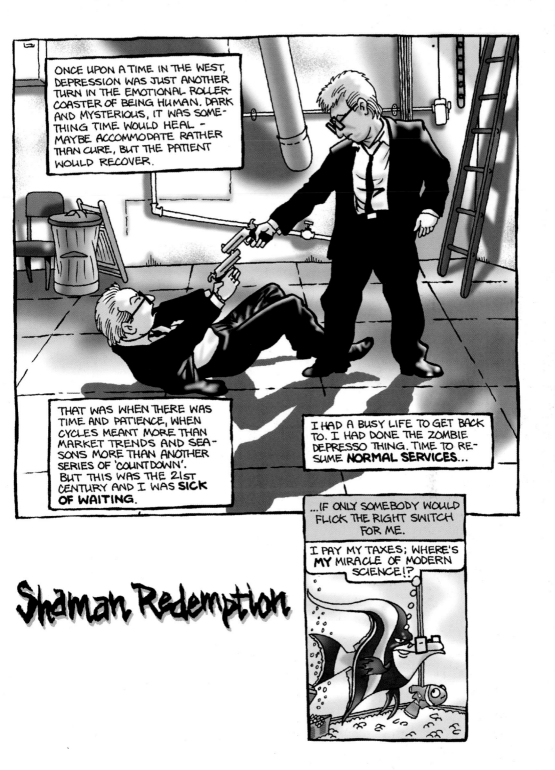

ONCE UPON A TIME IN THE WEST, DEPRESSION WAS JUST ANOTHER TURN IN THE EMOTIONAL ROLLER-COASTER OF BEING HUMAN. DARK AND MYSTERIOUS, IT WAS SOMETHING TIME WOULD HEAL - MAYBE ACCOMMODATE RATHER THAN CURE, BUT THE PATIENT WOULD RECOVER.

THAT WAS WHEN THERE WAS TIME AND PATIENCE, WHEN CYCLES MEANT MORE THAN MARKET TRENDS AND SEASONS MORE THAN ANOTHER SERIES OF 'COUNTDOWN'. BUT THIS WAS THE 21st CENTURY AND I WAS **SICK OF WAITING.**

I HAD A BUSY LIFE TO GET BACK TO. I HAD DONE THE ZOMBIE DEPRESSO THING. TIME TO RESUME **NORMAL SERVICES...**

...IF ONLY SOMEBODY WOULD FLICK THE RIGHT SWITCH FOR ME.

I PAY MY TAXES; WHERE'S **MY** MIRACLE OF MODERN SCIENCE!?

Shaman Redemption

IN THE 1700s I WOULD HAVE BEEN DIAGNOSED **INSANE** AND CONFINED TO A MADHOUSE, POSSIBLY MANACLED, CERTAINLY BEATEN FOR BEING 'IRASCIBLE'.

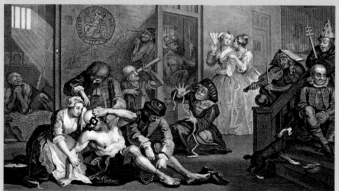

BLEEDINGS, PURGES, EMETICS AND NAUSEA INDUCING MERCURY WERE USED TO QUELL THE BEAST IN ME...

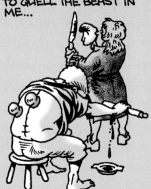

AND I SPENT WEEKS AT A TIME BEING DOWSED IN FREEZING WATER IN THAT MIRACLE OF MODERN SCIENCE, THE **TRANQUILISER CHAIR**.

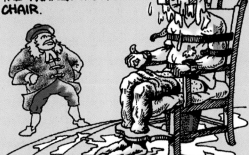

IN THE 1800s SCIENCE DECIDED MY SPAWN WOULD BE MORAL, INTELLECTUAL AND PHYSICAL **RETARDS**, SO I WAS CASTRATED. APPARENTLY THIS ALSO CRUSHED MY LIBIDO, RELIEVING ME OF A SOURCE OF TERRIBLE INNER TORMENT.

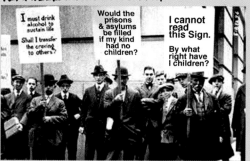

I must drink alcohol to sustain life

Shall I transfer the craving to others?

Would the prisons & asylums be filled if my kind had no children?

I cannot read this Sign.

By what right have I children?

(THE EUGENICS APPROACH ONLY LOST FAVOUR WHEN DOCTORS IN THE 1940s GOT A LITTLE CARRIED AWAY.)

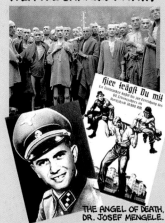

THE ANGEL OF DEATH, DR. JOSEF MENGELE.

IN THE EARLY 1900s I WAS FORCIBLY COMATOSED, CONVULSED (WHICH BROKE MY PELVIS) AND **ZAPPED** FOR MY OWN GOOD.

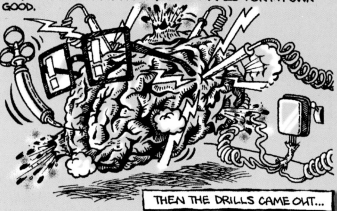

THEN THE DRILLS CAME OUT...

THE **PREFRONTAL LOBOTOMY** WORKED A TREAT, MIRACULOUSLY TRANSFORMING ME FROM ANIMAL TO VEGETABLE, BUT THE BLACK + DECKER APPROACH WAS A TOUGH SELL....

IN THE 1950s SCIENCE REVOLUTIONISED MAD MEDICINE BY CONCOCTING A PILL THAT DID THE JOB OF A DRILL.

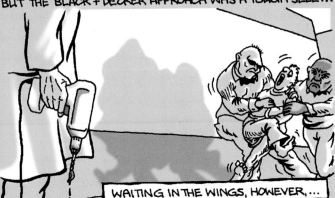

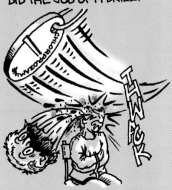

WAITING IN THE WINGS, HOWEVER, ...

SO BEGAN THE HIT AND MISS GAME OF TINKERING WITH MY CHEMISTRY. SO BEGAN THE RISE AND RISE OF DRUG COMPANIES TO WORLD DOMINATION OF MAD MEDICINE.

IN THE 1970s THE WORLD HEALTH ORGANISATION FOUND **64%** OF NUTTERS IN POOR COUNTRIES, WHERE THEY COULDN'T AFFORD MODERN MEDS, WERE DOING WELL FIVE YEARS ON. IN THE DRUG RICH NORTH, **65%** HAD SLIPPED BACKWARDS AND WERE NOW CHRONICALLY ILL.

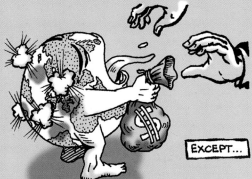

EXCEPT...

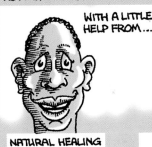

WITH A LITTLE HELP FROM...

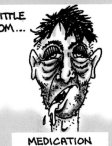

NATURAL HEALING

MEDICATION

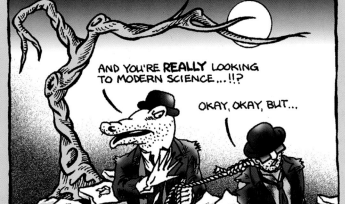

AND YOU'RE **REALLY** LOOKING TO MODERN SCIENCE...!!?

OKAY, OKAY, BUT...

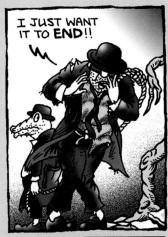

I JUST WANT IT TO **END**!!

MEANWHILE...

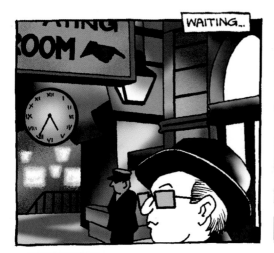

WAITING...

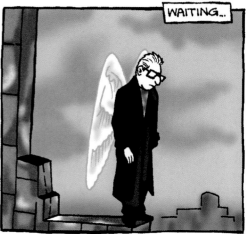

WAITING...

WAITING...

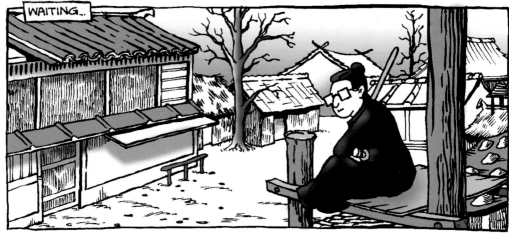

IN LIEU OF ANY ARM OF THE NATIONAL HEALTH SERVICE REACHING OUT A HELPING HAND, I TOOK MYSELF OFF TO A 'PERSONAL DEVELOPMENT COURSE'.

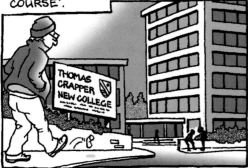

S'CUSE ME. WHAT ROOM FOR 'COPING WITH DEPRESSION'?

NOT A LOT, BY THE LOOK OF THINGS!

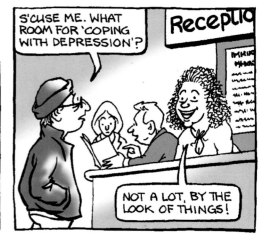

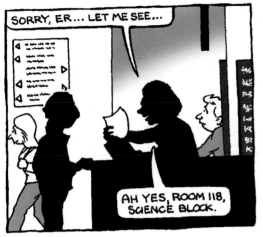

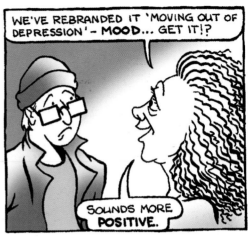

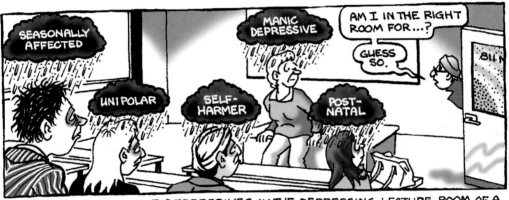

SO THERE WE WERE, FIVE DEPRESSIVES IN THE DEPRESSING LECTURE ROOM OF A DEPRESSING F.E. COLLEGE WITH A LECTURER WHO WARNED US STRAIGHT OFF THAT DEPRESSION IS DEPRESSINGLY DIFFICULT TO UNDERSTAND.

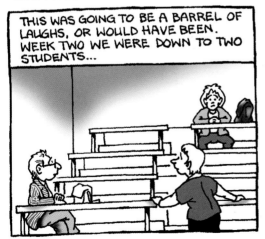

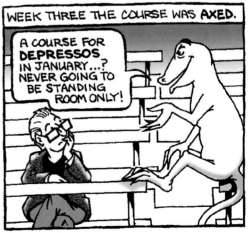

THE THIRD MONDAY IN JANUARY IS OFFICIALLY RECOGNISED BY THE MEDICAL PROFESSION AS THE DAY ON WHICH MORE U.K. CITIZENS WAKE UP DEPRESSED THAN ANY OTHER. THE REALITY OF ANOTHER GRINDING YEAR KICKS IN, THE HORROR OF THE CHRISTMAS CREDIT CARD BILL BITES, THE MISERY OF ANOTHER RAIN-LASHED DAY DAWNS ...

SUFFICE TO SAY, IT'S ONE **BUMMER** OF A DAY IN A BUMMER OF A **MONTH**.

BY FAIR MEANS OR FOUL, MORE PEOPLE **SNUFF IT** IN JANUARY THAN IN ANY OTHER MONTH.

ON THE WAY HOME FROM THE COLLEGE SOMETHING **FREAKY** HAPPENED.

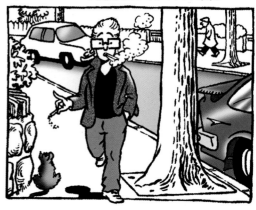

MY LEGS GREW HEAVY AND FEET BEGAN TO DRAG,

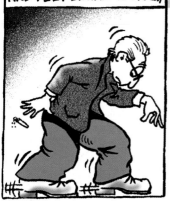

HUGE PUFFBALLS WELLED UP BENEATH MY EYES,

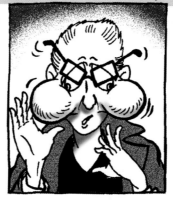

AND CASCADES OF UN-CONTROLLABLE TEARS FLOODED FORTH!

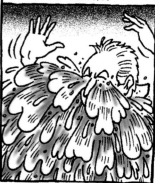

OUR POSTMAN FOUND ME.

YOU ALRIGHT, MR. FREEMAN?

ER...

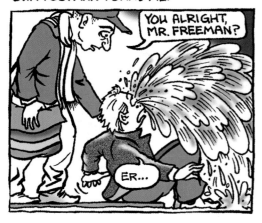

WHAT COULD I SAY? TIGHT UNDER-PANTS? RAGING TOOTHACHE? POST-TRAUMATIC CHRISTMAS DISORDER?

MR. FREEMAN?

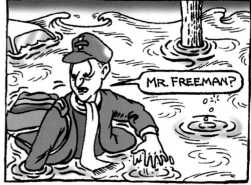

168

IT WASN'T THE FIRST TIME I'D BEEN **MUGGED** BY THE CROCODILES. OFF AND ON, THEY'D BEEN SPRINGING SURPRISE ATTACKS FOR DECADES. EVEN IF THEY DID STRIKE WITH THE **STEALTH** OF ODYSSEUS, I THOUGHT IT A **GOOD SIGN**, AS IN, "HEY, I'M IN TOUCH WITH MY EMOTIONS!"

IN RETROSPECT, I'VE BALLED MY EYES OUT OVER SOME PRETTY STRANGE THINGS, LIKE ...

CYCLING IN WINTER PAST THE GLOW FROM A SITTING ROOM WHEREIN I PICTURED A FAMILY, COSY AND CONTENTED.

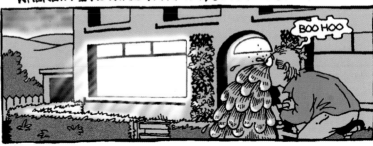

BOO HOO

GLEN COE, 5:00 AM, BATHED IN MIST, WARMED BY DELICATE RAYS, BRACED FOR A STORM.

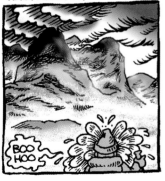

BOO HOO

ON FIRST HEARING SMETANA'S **'MA VAST'**, GRANDPA MIKLOS' FAVOURITE PIECE.

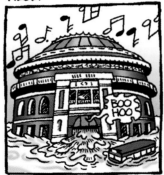

BOO HOO

FINAL REEL OF 'FINDING NEVERLAND'. (OKAY, MAYBE THAT'S NOT SO STRANGE.)

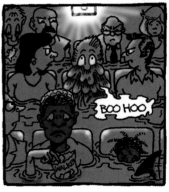

BOO HOO

BUT IT WASN'T ONLY EXTREME SOBBING THAT HIJACKED ME. TAKE MY REACTIONS TO...

THE DEATH OF DIANA, PRINCESS OF WALES...

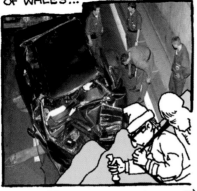

AND THE ATTACK ON NEW YORK

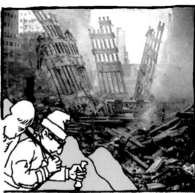

(I WAS...   IN THE TORRIDONS AT THE TIME)   IN THE EUROPAS AT THE TIME)

IN BOTH CASES IT WAS **THREE DAYS** BEFORE I HEARD THE NEWS.

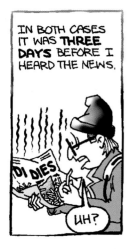

DI DIES

UH?

EACH TIME I WALKED OUT OF THE MOUNTAINS INTO A WORLD TAKEN LEAVE OF ITS SENSES.

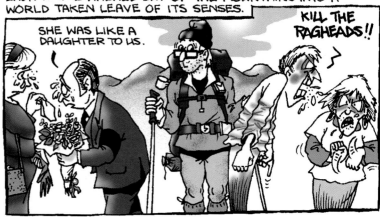

SHE WAS LIKE A DAUGHTER TO US.

KILL THE RAGHEADS!!

BY THE TIME I CAUGHT UP, INTER-FLORA HAD REPAVED THE MALL AND THE PRESIDENT REDEFINED THE MIDDLE EAST.

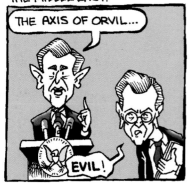

THE AXIS OF ORVIL...

EVIL!

MY REACTION...?

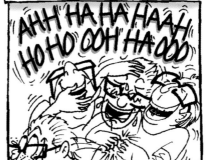

AHH HA HA HAAH HO HO OOH HA OOO

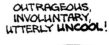

OUTRAGEOUS, INVOLUNTARY, UTTERLY **UNCOOL**!

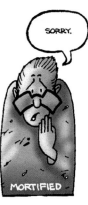

SORRY.

MORTIFIED

WERE THESE THE RANT-INGS OF A CARTOONIST **AWOL** FOR THE BIGGEST MEDIA FESTS OF THE MODERN ERA...?

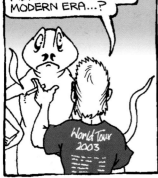

World Tour 2003

OR THE **HYSTERICS** OF SOMEONE AWARE OF GREATER TRAGEDIES IN THE WORLD DESERVING OUR SYMPATHIES...?

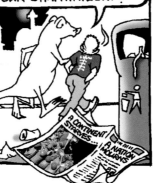

A CONTINENT STARVES...

A NATION MOURNS

OR WAS I SIMPLY SUFFER-ING FROM INVOLUNTARY EMOTIONAL EXPRESSION DISORDER?

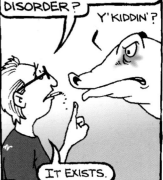

Y'KIDDIN'?

IT EXISTS.

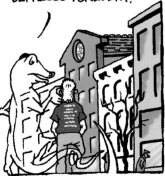

SO WHAT, YOU'VE BEEN A DEPRESSO FOREVER!?

US **IEED**ERS PREFER 'EMOTIONALLY DYSCONTROLLED'.

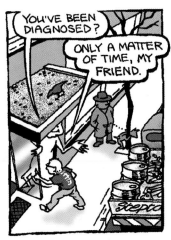

YOU'VE BEEN DIAGNOSED?

ONLY A MATTER OF TIME, MY FRIEND.

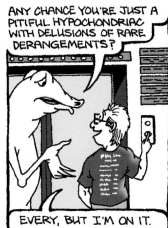

ANY CHANCE YOU'RE JUST A PITIFUL HYPOCHONDRIAC WITH DELUSIONS OF RARE DERANGEMENTS?

EVERY, BUT I'M ON IT.

I HAD CALLED IN A FAVOUR FROM A PAL, A STRESS MANAGEMENT SOMETHING-OR-OTHER.

OKAY, TOM, CLOSE YOUR EYES, RELAX, PICTURE ANY OBJECT IN THE ROOM.

I NEEDED SOMETHING STRONGER THAN THE PILLS TO RELAX ME - AN ANXIETY BUSTING EXERCISE, A RUBBER BAND TO TWANG...

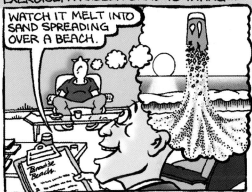

WATCH IT MELT INTO SAND SPREADING OVER A BEACH.

"YOU ARE ON **PARADISE BEACH**. FEEL THE WARM WHITE SAND, HEAR THE SEA LAPPING, THE PALMS RUSTLING, SMELL THE FACTOR 50 SIZZLING."

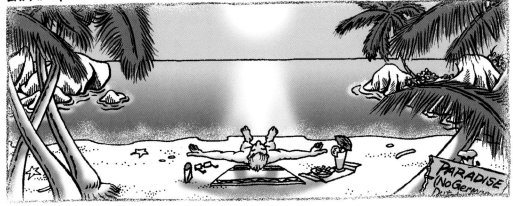

"THE SUN PENETRATES YOUR BODY, WARMS THE DARKEST RECESS, RELAXES EVERY MUSCLE AND TENDON."

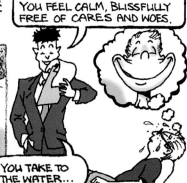

YOU FEEL CALM, BLISSFULLY FREE OF CARES AND WOES.

YOU TAKE TO THE WATER...

"FEEL THE SOUTH SEA LAPPING AGAINST YOU, STIMULATING, INVIGORATING. YOU FEEL **STRONG**..."

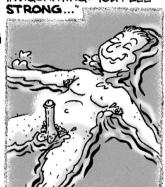

THUS HE **PILED ON** PARADISE BEACH FOR HALF AN HOUR BEFORE...

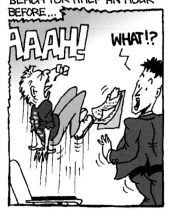

AAAH!

WHAT!?

TSUNAMI!!!

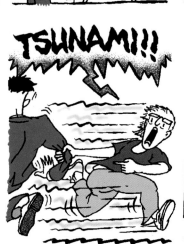

TSUNAMI?

RUN!

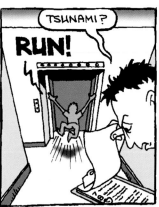

SEEMS I HAD AN AVERSION TO AVERSION THERAPY.

I WENT BACK TO MY MUSIC AND WAITING.

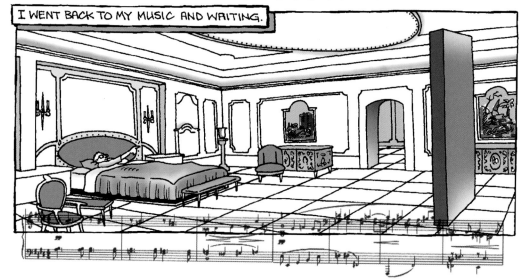

IF NEEDS MUST, I CAN BE A **CONSUMMATE WAITER.**

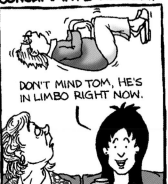

DON'T MIND TOM, HE'S IN LIMBO RIGHT NOW.

AGED EIGHT, I MISSED MY FIRST RAIL CONNECTION...

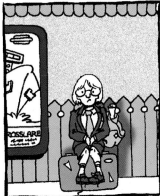

WHICH MEANT A **TWO DAY** WAIT AT HEATHROW FOR ANOTHER FLIGHT OUT TO VISIT THE PARENTS.

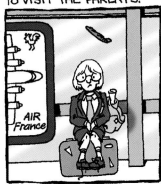

AIR France

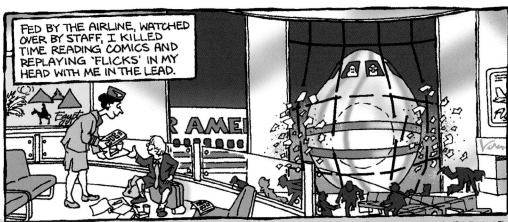

FED BY THE AIRLINE, WATCHED OVER BY STAFF, I KILLED TIME READING COMICS AND REPLAYING 'FLICKS' IN MY HEAD WITH ME IN THE LEAD.

DURING ONE SUCH SOJOURN IN LIMBOLAND I DEVELOPED **FREEMAN'S THEORY OF CRITICAL BOREDOM,** WHICH STATED...

THERE IS NOWHERE ON THIS PLANET AN ACTIVE IMAGINATION CAN BECOME BORED.

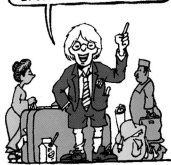

ERGO, ONLY BORING PEOPLE GET BORED (LONG TERM HOSTAGES EXCEPTED).

TALK TO ME.

I HADN'T ACCOUNTED FOR DEPRESSOS.

I MEAN, I **KNOW** HOW TO WAIT, BUT...

YOU'VE REACH-ED **CRITICAL THRESHOLD**?

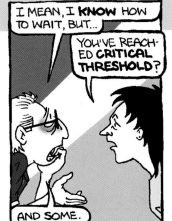

AND SOME.

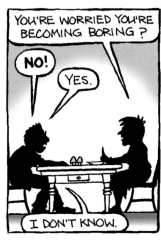

YOU'RE WORRIED YOU'RE BECOMING BORING?

NO!

YES.

I DON'T KNOW.

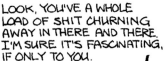
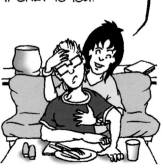
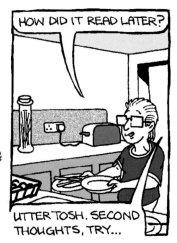

LOOK, YOU'VE A WHOLE LOAD OF SHIT CHURNING AWAY IN THERE AND THERE. I'M SURE IT'S FASCINATING, IF ONLY TO YOU.

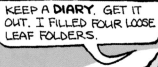
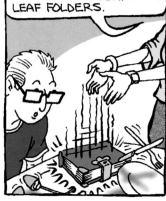

KEEP A **DIARY**. GET IT OUT. I FILLED FOUR LOOSE LEAF FOLDERS.

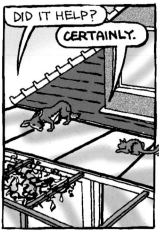

DID IT HELP?

CERTAINLY.

HOW DID IT READ LATER?

UTTER TOSH. SECOND THOUGHTS, TRY...

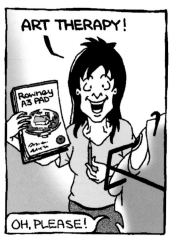

ART THERAPY!

Rowney A3 PAD

OH, PLEASE!

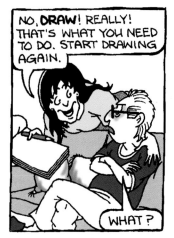

NO, **DRAW**! REALLY! THAT'S WHAT YOU NEED TO DO. START DRAWING AGAIN.

WHAT?

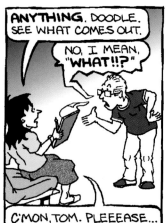

ANYTHING. DOODLE. SEE WHAT COMES OUT.

NO, I MEAN, "**WHAT!!?**"

C'MON, TOM. PLEEEASE...

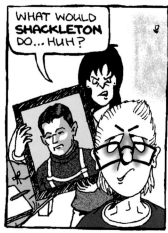

WHAT WOULD **SHACKLETON** DO... HUH?

174

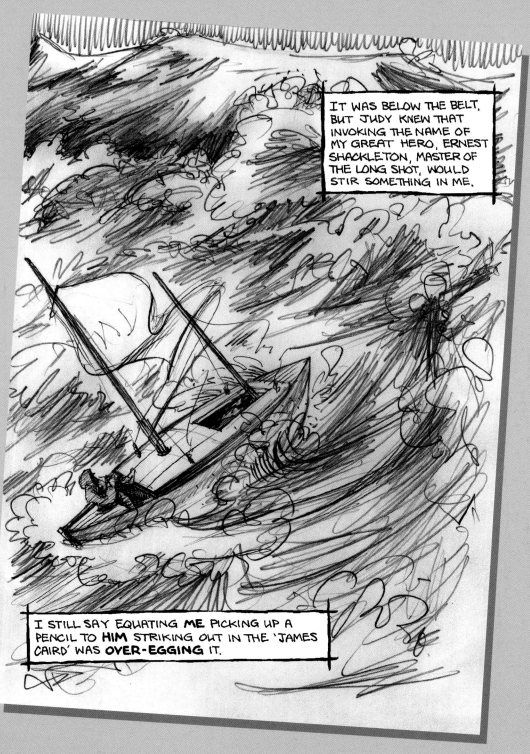

IT WAS BELOW THE BELT, BUT JUDY KNEW THAT INVOKING THE NAME OF MY GREAT HERO, ERNEST SHACKLETON, MASTER OF THE LONG SHOT, WOULD STIR SOMETHING IN ME.

I STILL SAY EQUATING **ME** PICKING UP A PENCIL TO **HIM** STRIKING OUT IN THE 'JAMES CAIRD' WAS **OVER-EGGING** IT.

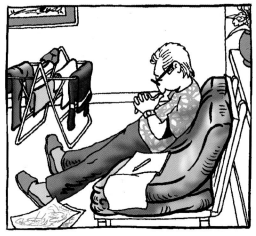

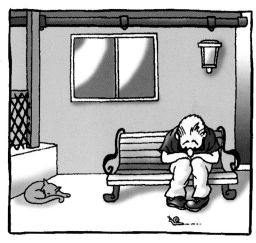

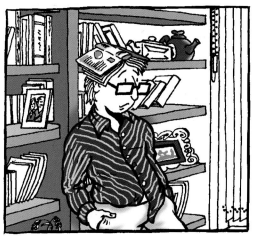

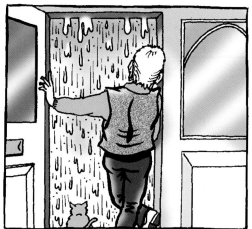

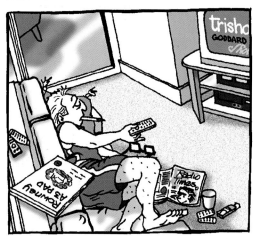

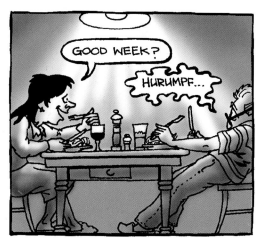

PEOPLE HAD BEEN ON AT ME,

NONE MORE SO THAN JUDY.

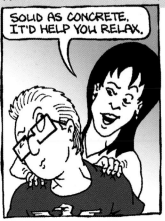

SOLID AS CONCRETE. IT'D HELP YOU RELAX.

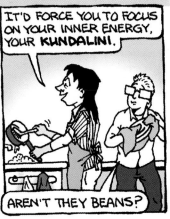

IT'D FORCE YOU TO FOCUS ON YOUR INNER ENERGY, YOUR **KUNDALINI**.

AREN'T THEY BEANS?

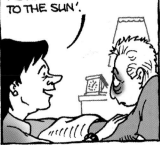

...HALF AN HOUR EACH MORNING WITH 'SALUTE TO THE SUN'.

FOR A QUIET LIFE AS MUCH AS TO TRY SOMETHING EVERY-BODY SAID WOULD BE BENE-FICIAL, I TOOK UP **YOGA**...

...AN ACTIVITY THAT REQU-IRES MORE ARTIFICIAL AIDS THAN STEPHEN HAWKINS.

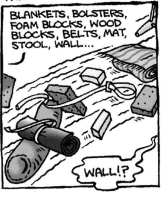

BLANKETS, BOLSTERS, FOAM BLOCKS, WOOD BLOCKS, BELTS, MAT, STOOL, WALL....

WALL!?

JUST CARRYING ALL THE CLOBBER TO THE CLASS WAS ENOUGH TO PUT A BLOKE'S BACK OUT.

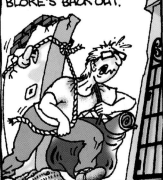

AS FOR THE EXERCISES, THEY WEREN'T CALLED POSES FOR NOTHING.

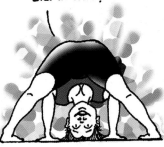

DOES MY BUM LOOK BIG IN THIS?

THE ONLY TIME I BROKE INTO A SWEAT WAS WHEN CALLED UPON TO...

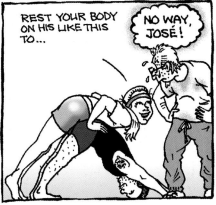

REST YOUR BODY ON HIS LIKE THIS TO...

NO WAY, JOSÉ!

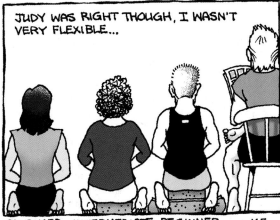

JUDY WAS RIGHT THOUGH, I WASN'T VERY FLEXIBLE...

ADVANCED   INTERMEDIATE BEGINNER   ME.

177

BUT HOW ANY OF THIS WAS SUPPOSED TO IMPROVE MY STATE OF MIND...?

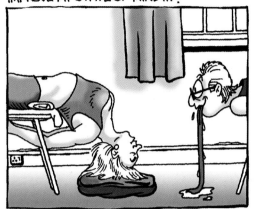

THE RELAXATION BIT AT THE END WAS PLAIN EMBARRASSING!

DEEP BREATHS, TOM...

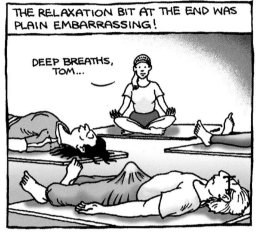

YOU DIDN'T RATE IT?

IT'S FINE FOR MOUSE-PUSHERS OF A CERTAIN AGE WITH THE ENERGY RESERVES OF A **STUFFED CAT.**

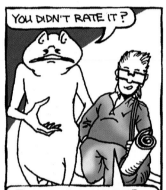

YOU WON'T BE GOING BACK THEN?

YOU KIDDING!!? LIVE SOFT-CORE AT THREE QUID AN HOUR...

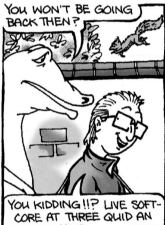

WONDERFUL TO HEAR YOU'RE EMBRACING THE YOGIC JOURNEY TO INNER PEACE AND SPIRITUAL HARMONY WITH SUCH VIGOUR.

......

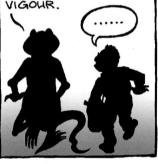

ORIGINALLY A PHILOSOPHY, THE FIRST YOGA POSES WERE DEVISED BY INDIAN SAGES LOOKING FOR A COMFY POSITION TO WHILE AWAY THEIR LIVES IN MEDIT-ATION.

THE AIM WAS TO CALM THE CHAOS OF **CONFLICTING IMPULSES** (A PAIN IN THE BUTT) **AND THOUGHTS** ("SOD THIS FOR A GAME OF MARBLES!") THAT GOT IN THE WAY OF ACHIEVING **COSMIC ENLIGHTEN-MENT.**

IT STILL IS THE AIM THOUGH, TYPICALLY, THE WEST CHANGED THE BEARING TO **SELF** ENLIGHTENMENT. SO YOGA IS NOW A STRESS-BUSTER FOR THE CHATTERATI.

2,000 YEARS AGO THE SAGES ATTRIBUTED MENTAL ILLNESS TO FIVE ENERGY SAPPING **SORROWS** THAT THROW YOUR MENTAL, PHYSICAL AND SPIRITUAL EQUILIBRIUM INTO A FLAT SPIN.

YOGA EXERCISES OR POSES (ASANAS) STIMULATE THE BLOOD FLOW, WHICH REGENERATES THE NERVES THAT STIMULATE THE BRAIN WHICH CONTROLS OUR MENTAL AND PHYSICAL FUNCTIONS.

BUT THE **MIND** ISN'T HOUSED IN THE HEAD, ACCORDING TO THE SAGES, IT IS EVERYWHERE, LATENT, ELUSIVE, FLITTING AROUND BETWEEN OUTER SKIN AND INNER BEING.

FLITTING WITH IT ARE THE INTELLECT, EMOTIONS, VITAL ENERGY, WILL POWER, CONSCIENCE AND SENSE OF SELF THAT MAKES US AN **INDIVIDUAL**. TOGETHER THEY ARE TEAM SOUL, POWERED BY THEIR OWN EQUALLY ELUSIVE SOURCES OF ENERGY, THE **CHAKRAS**.

THE CHAKRAS DON'T PHYSICALLY EXIST. THEY ARE PICTURED AS SEVEN COILS MOORED ALONG THE SPINE AND WIRED TO EVERY CORNER OF THE BODY BY A NETWORK OF CONDUITS (NADIS) WHICH ALSO DON'T PHYSICALLY EXIST.

COILED AND UNCOILED, THE CHAKRAS DRIVE OPPOSING EMOTIONS. ENERGY TRAPPED IN THE MAIPURAKA CHAKRA FUELS OUR FEARS. AS THE CHAKRA UNCOILS, THE ENERGY RELEASED INDUCES CALM. DEPRESSOS ARE BURDENED WITH A MESS OF SCREWED-UP CHAKRAS THAT YOGA CAN UNWIND, LIBERATING SPIRITUAL ENERGY FOR TEAM SOUL.

The Illuminated Self

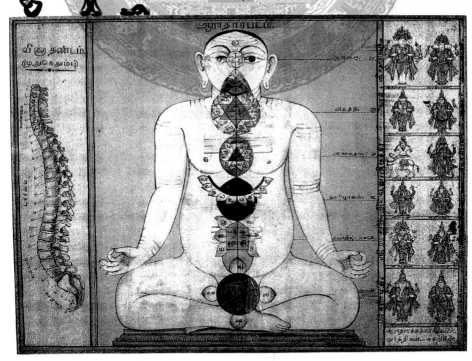

BECAUSE IT SEEKS TO INTEGRATE AND BALANCE UP **HEAD, HEART** AND **HAND**, EVERY TOM, DICK AND SALLY IN MENTAL HEALTH WHO ISN'T A RAGING CHRISTIAN NOW RECOMMENDS YOGA.

'CHRISPIES' RUN A MILE FROM ANYTHING PEDDLING SPIRITUAL ENLIGHTENMENT **NOT** IN A HABIT OR CASSOCK. PLUS, OF COURSE, THE ORIGINS OF YOGA ARE ROOTED WAY TOO CLOSE TO THE AXIS OF EVIL.

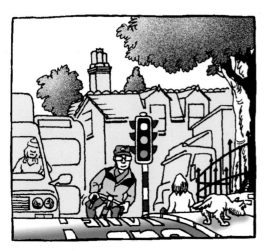

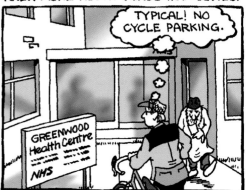

18 MONTHS AFTER BEING DIAGNOSED I FINALLY GOT TO SEE SOMEBODY WHO KNEW MORE ABOUT MINDS THAN BODIES.

TYPICAL! NO CYCLE PARKING.

GREENWOOD Health Centre

NHS

HE WENT BY THE TITLE 'NURSE PRACTIONER IN MENTAL HEALTH'.

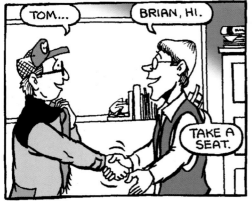

TOM...

BRIAN, HI.

TAKE A SEAT.

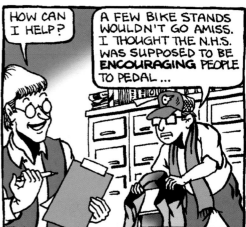

HOW CAN I HELP?

A FEW BIKE STANDS WOULDN'T GO AMISS. I THOUGHT THE N.H.S. WAS SUPPOSED TO BE **ENCOURAGING** PEOPLE TO PEDAL ...

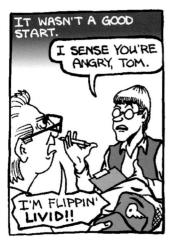

IT WASN'T A GOOD START.

I SENSE YOU'RE ANGRY, TOM.

I'M FLIPPIN' **LIVID!!**

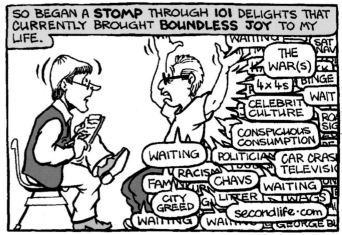

SO BEGAN A **STOMP** THROUGH **101** DELIGHTS THAT CURRENTLY BROUGHT **BOUNDLESS JOY** TO MY LIFE.

WAITING · SAT NAV · THE WAR(S) · BINGE · 4x4s · WAIT · CELEBRITY CULTURE · CONSPICUOUS CONSUMPTION · WAITING · POLITICIANS · CAR CRASH · TELEVISION · RACISM · CHAVS · WAITING · FAMILY · CITY GREED · LITTER · TWIGS · secondlife.com · WAITING · WAITING · GEORGE B

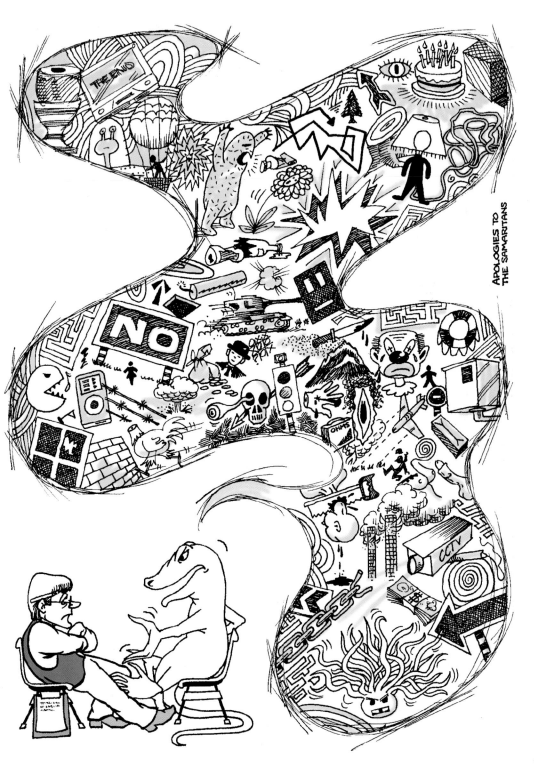

APOLOGIES TO THE SAMARITANS

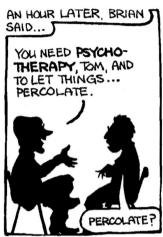

AN HOUR LATER, BRIAN SAID...

YOU NEED **PSYCHO-THERAPY**, TOM, AND TO LET THINGS... PERCOLATE.

PERCOLATE?

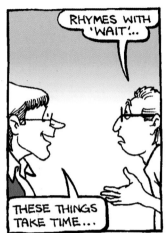

RHYMES WITH 'WAIT'...

THESE THINGS TAKE TIME...

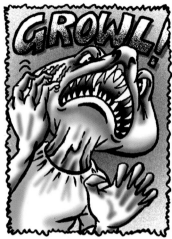

GROWL!

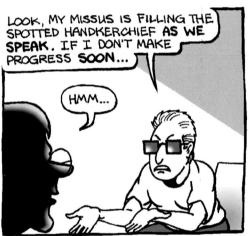

LOOK, MY MISSUS IS FILLING THE SPOTTED HANDKERCHIEF **AS WE SPEAK**. IF I DON'T MAKE PROGRESS **SOON**...

HMM...

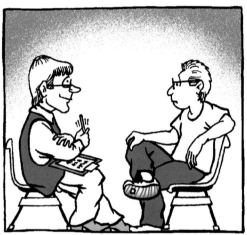

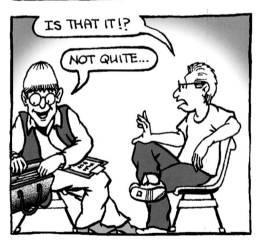

IS THAT IT!?

NOT QUITE...

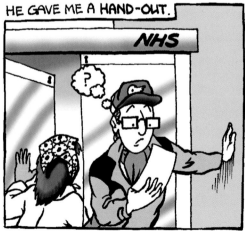

HE GAVE ME A **HAND-OUT**.

NHS

?

182

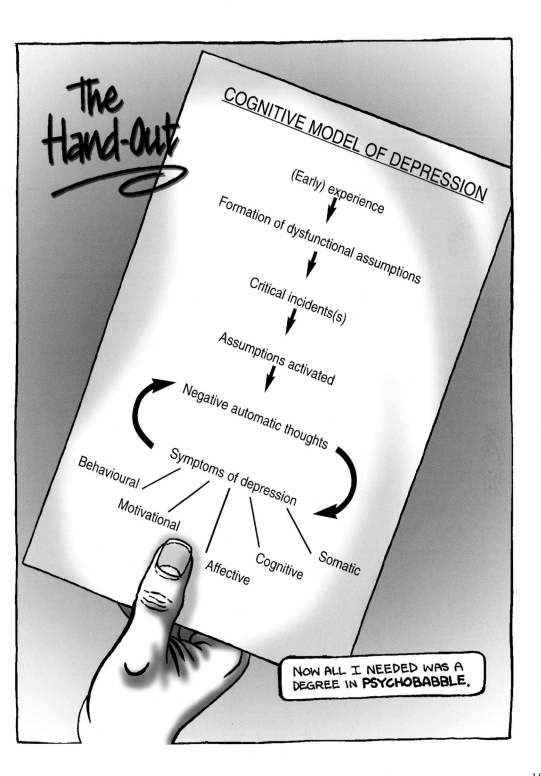

183

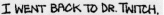
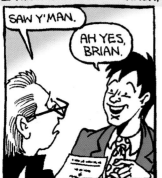
I WENT BACK TO DR. TWITCH.

SAW Y'MAN.

AH YES, BRIAN.

GAVE ME THIS, SAID I NEEDED PSYCHOTHERAPY.

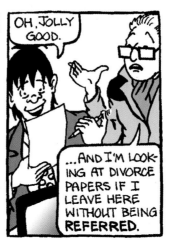
OH, JOLLY GOOD.

...AND I'M LOOKING AT DIVORCE PAPERS IF I LEAVE HERE WITHOUT BEING REFERRED.

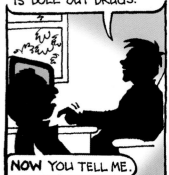
CAN'T HELP YOU, OLD SON. BRIAN'S THE GATEKEEPER. ALL I CAN DO IS DOLE OUT DRUGS.

NOW YOU TELL ME.

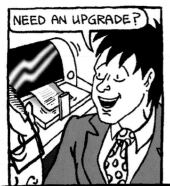
NEED AN UPGRADE?

(DRUG No. 4 = SERTRALINE. ANOTHER SSRI, GOOD FOR OCD AND PTSD.*)

UNLESS THEY'VE A TOTAL WACKO ON THEIR HANDS, GPs IN THE U.K. CANNOT ACCESS MENTAL HEALTH SERVICES DIRECTLY. IT'S THE OLD PHYSICAL-MENTAL DIVIDE. GPs PROVIDE PRIMARY CARE. HEAD CASES REQUIRE SECONDARY CARE. COMMON OR GARDEN PSYCHOS HAVE TO BE REFERRED THROUGH A BRIAN WHO ADMINISTERS HAND-OUTS AND PRESCRIBES 'PERCOLATION'.

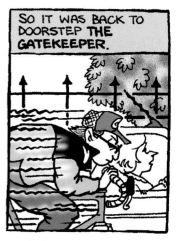
SO IT WAS BACK TO DOORSTEP THE GATEKEEPER.

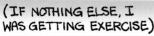
(IF NOTHING ELSE, I WAS GETTING EXERCISE)

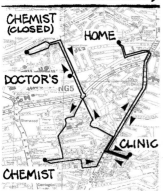
CHEMIST (CLOSED)

HOME

DOCTOR'S

NG5

CLINIC

CHEMIST

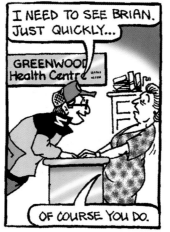
I NEED TO SEE BRIAN. JUST QUICKLY...

GREENWOOD Health Centre

OF COURSE YOU DO.

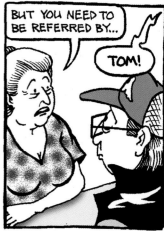
BUT YOU NEED TO BE REFERRED BY...

TOM!

* OCD - OBSESSIVE COMPULSIVE DISORDER
PTSD - POST-TRAUMATIC STRESS DISORDER

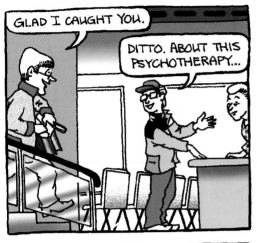

GLAD I CAUGHT YOU.

DITTO. ABOUT THIS PSYCHOTHERAPY...

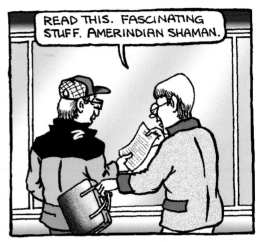

READ THIS. FASCINATING STUFF. AMERINDIAN SHAMAN.

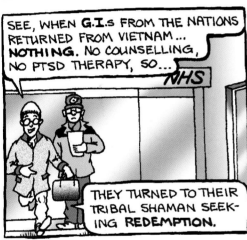

SEE, WHEN **G.I.**s FROM THE NATIONS RETURNED FROM VIETNAM... **NOTHING.** NO COUNSELLING, NO PTSD THERAPY, SO...

NHS

THEY TURNED TO THEIR TRIBAL SHAMAN SEEKING **REDEMPTION.**

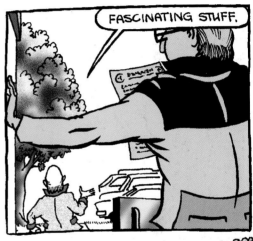

FASCINATING STUFF.

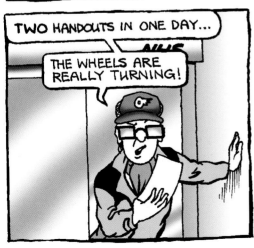

TWO HANDOUTS IN ONE DAY...

NHS

THE WHEELS ARE REALLY TURNING!

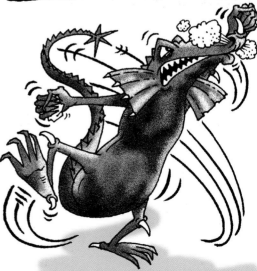

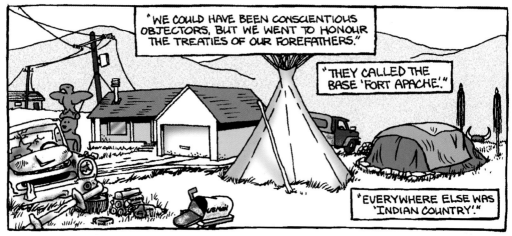

"WE COULD HAVE BEEN CONSCIENTIOUS OBJECTORS, BUT WE WENT TO HONOUR THE TREATIES OF OUR FOREFATHERS."

"THEY CALLED THE BASE 'FORT APACHE.'"

"EVERYWHERE ELSE WAS 'INDIAN COUNTRY'."

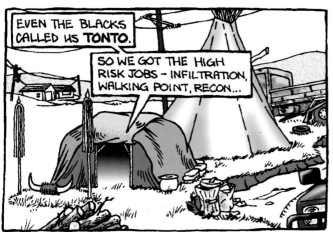

EVEN THE BLACKS CALLED US **TONTO**.

SO WE GOT THE HIGH RISK JOBS – INFILTRATION, WALKING POINT, RECON...

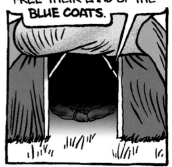

WE SAW THE GOOKS WERE THE SAME COLOUR AS US – RED, BUT NOT **COMMIES**. THEY WERE FIGHTING TO FREE THEIR LAND OF THE **BLUE COATS**.

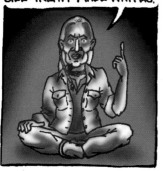

THE GREAT WHITE CHIEFS WERE UP TO THEIR OLD TRICKS AGAIN. THEY NEVER HONOURED A SIN-GLE TREATY MADE WITH US.

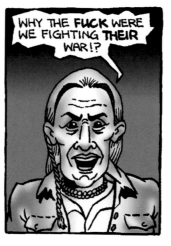

WHY THE **FUCK** WERE WE FIGHTING **THEIR** WAR!?

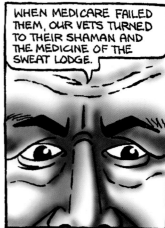

WHEN MEDICARE FAILED THEM, OUR VETS TURNED TO THEIR SHAMAN AND THE MEDICINE OF THE SWEAT LODGE.

186

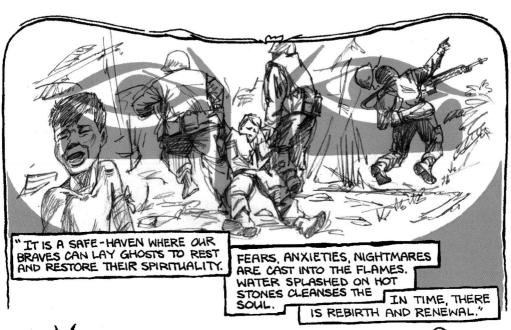

"IT IS A SAFE-HAVEN WHERE OUR BRAVES CAN LAY GHOSTS TO REST AND RESTORE THEIR SPIRITUALITY.

FEARS, ANXIETIES, NIGHTMARES ARE CAST INTO THE FLAMES. WATER SPLASHED ON HOT STONES CLEANSES THE SOUL.

IN TIME, THERE IS REBIRTH AND RENEWAL."

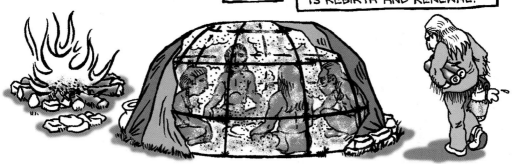

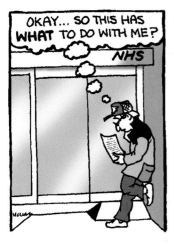

OKAY... SO THIS HAS **WHAT** TO DO WITH ME?

NHS

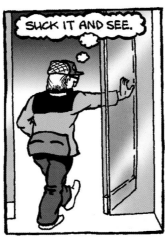

SUCK IT AND SEE.

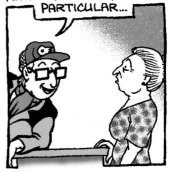

HELLO AGAIN. DO YOU KNOW IF THERE'S AN AMERICAN INDIAN SHAMAN PRACTISING IN TOWN? NAVAJO, APACHE, I'M NOT PARTICULAR...

I HADN'T THE FOGGIEST WHERE BRIAN WAS STEERING ME. IN THIS COUNTRY, A SWEAT LODGE WOULD BE STIFF WITH 'GUARDIAN' READERS SEEKING REDEMPTION AFTER A WEEK STICKING IT TO THE PLEBS.

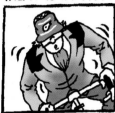

WHAT THE HELL WAS REDEMPTION ANYWAY, AND WHY DID I NEED IT?

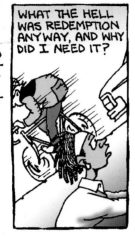

I ASKED SOMEONE WITH A SHOE-IN TO THE **HIGHEST AUTHORITY.**

IT'S THE RESTORATION OF MANKIND FROM THE BONDAGE OF SIN TO THE LIBERTY OF THE CHILDREN OF GOD THROUGH THE SATISFACTIONS AND MERITS OF CHRIST OUR LORD, OKAY?

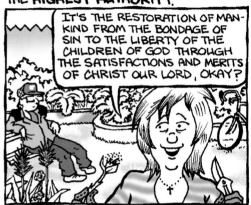

SOOO... I'M LOOKING FOR THREE NAILS AND A COUPLE OF JOISTS?

CHRIST BEAT YOU TO IT.

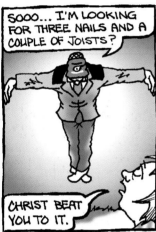

GOD GAVE HIS ONLY BEGOTTEN SON FOR YOUR SINS.

WAS I AROUND THEN?

WHAT SINS?

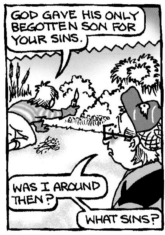

NO, DON'T TELL ME!!

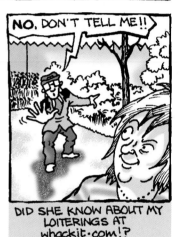

DID SHE KNOW ABOUT MY LOITERINGS AT whackit·com!?

SEEMS I NEED DELIVERANCE FROM MY SINS, SAVING FROM EVIL.

LIKE YOU'RE HAROLD SHIPMAN OR SUMMINT?

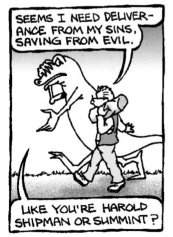

I DID ONCE DROWN A LITTER OF KITTENS.

C'MON, YOUR GREATEST SIN IS BEING HETEROSEXUAL AND INTO **MUSICALS.**

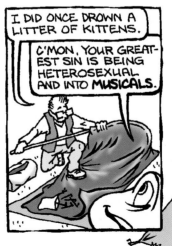

AN INTENSE PERIOD OF SELF REFLECTION WAS EVIDENTLY IN ORDER. I SWORE VOWS OF SILENCE AND ABSTINENCE. (EXCEPT AT MEALTIMES), AND WENT INTO **RETREAT.**

I'VE SINNED ALL MY LIFE. IT'S HOW I'VE **SURVIVED**, F'CHRISSAKE. GOOD SINS AND BAD.

BAD SINS BITE ME IN THE ARSE SOMEWHERE DOWN THE LINE, ALWAYS HAVE.

THE GOOD THING ABOUT MY BAD SINS IS THAT I WISE UP FAST. THE BAD THING IS THAT THEY KEEP COOKING UP NEW BAD SINS FOR ME TO CHOKE ON.

THERE IS A GOD, DAMMIT, BUT I'VE CLEARED THE SLATE, HAVEN'T I?

WAY I SEE IT, A LOT OF BAD SINS ARE ACTUALLY GOOD SINS.

SURE, I'VE COMMITTED THEM; I'VE ENJOYED 'EM AND GOT AWAY WITH THE BUGGERS.

IN FACT, **NOT** TAKING FULL ADVANTAGE WOULD HAVE BEEN A BAD SIN IN MY BOOK.

BUT WHAT WAS THE SIN I COMMITTED THAT WAS SO HEINOUS, SO EVIL GOD RIPPED MY SOUL OUT AND SENT ME CRAWLING TO SHAMAN BRIAN?

WHAT WAS THE WAR CRIME THAT TRIGGERED MY PTSD?

AS FAR AS I CAN RECALL, I'VE BEEN ONE OF THE GOOD GUYS, ALL SINS CONSIDERED...

BUT I ONLY REMEMBER BACK TO WHEN I WAS EIGHT.

WAS THAT **IT**!!?

WAS **THAT** WHY MY PARENTS WALKED AWAY FROM ME?

SOMETIME BETWEEN FIRST BUGGY AND FIRST BIKE I DID SOMETHING TRULY APPALLING.

THE BOARDING SCHOOL WAS RETRIBUTION...

CHRIST, I MUST HAVE **MURDERED** SOMEBODY!!!

189

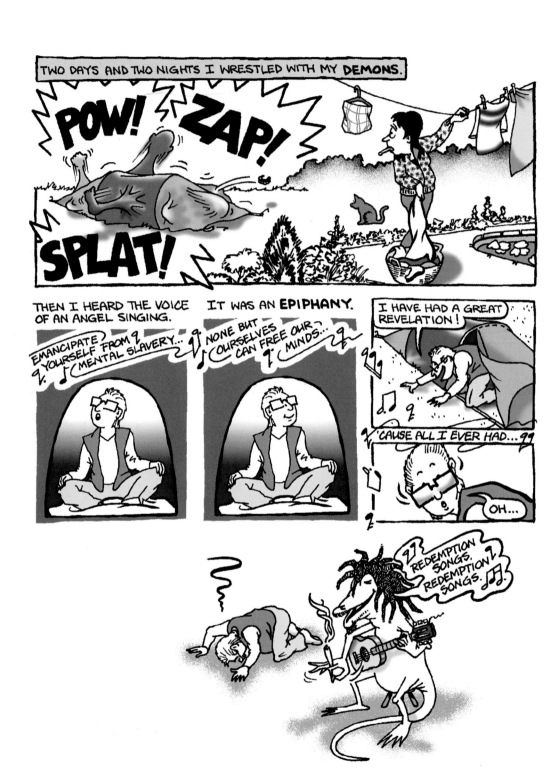

190

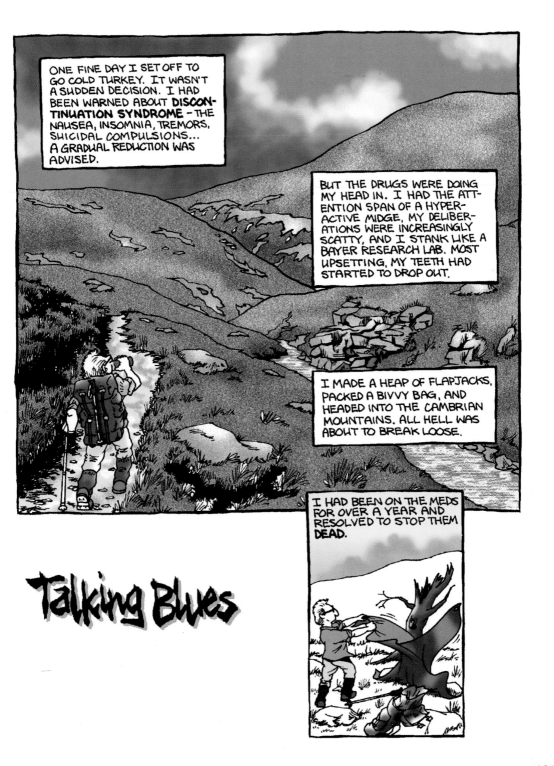

ONE FINE DAY I SET OFF TO GO COLD TURKEY. IT WASN'T A SUDDEN DECISION. I HAD BEEN WARNED ABOUT **DISCONTINUATION SYNDROME** – THE NAUSEA, INSOMNIA, TREMORS, SUICIDAL COMPULSIONS... A GRADUAL REDUCTION WAS ADVISED.

BUT THE DRUGS WERE DOING MY HEAD IN. I HAD THE ATTENTION SPAN OF A HYPERACTIVE MIDGE, MY DELIBERATIONS WERE INCREASINGLY SCATTY, AND I STANK LIKE A BAYER RESEARCH LAB. MOST UPSETTING, MY TEETH HAD STARTED TO DROP OUT.

I MADE A HEAP OF FLAPJACKS, PACKED A BIVVY BAG, AND HEADED INTO THE CAMBRIAN MOUNTAINS. ALL HELL WAS ABOUT TO BREAK LOOSE.

I HAD BEEN ON THE MEDS FOR OVER A YEAR AND RESOLVED TO STOP THEM **DEAD**.

Talking Blues

191

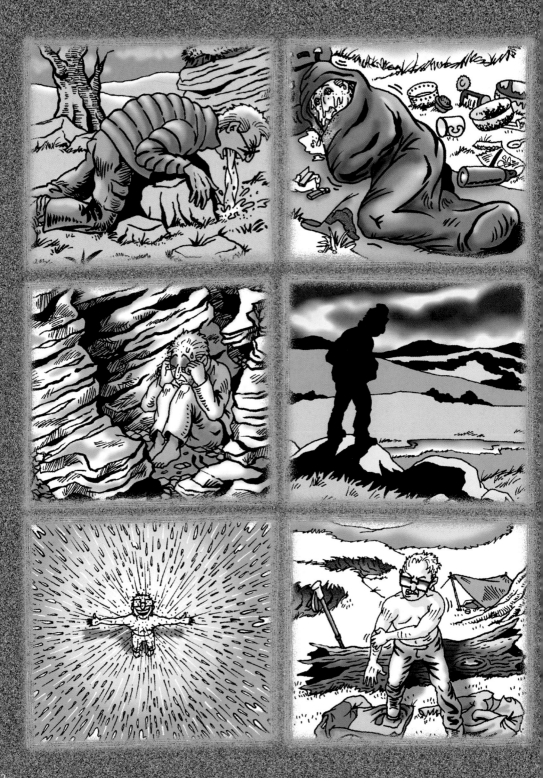

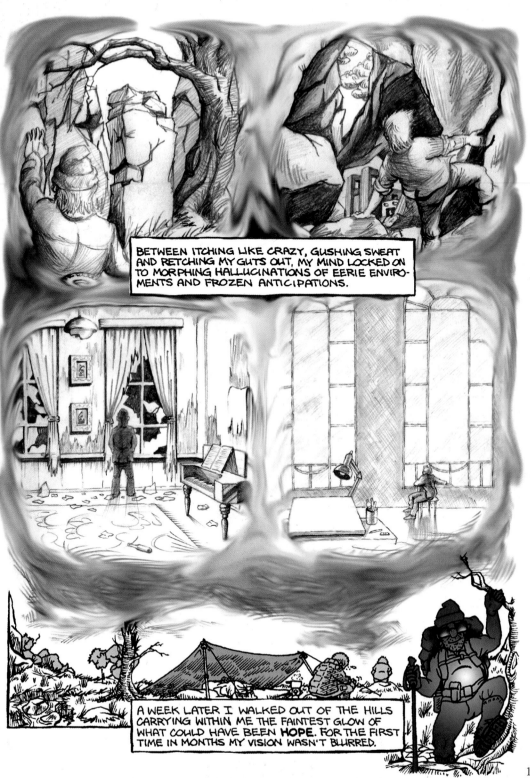

BETWEEN ITCHING LIKE CRAZY, GUSHING SWEAT AND RETCHING MY GUTS OUT, MY MIND LOCKED ON TO MORPHING HALLUCINATIONS OF EERIE ENVIROMENTS AND FROZEN ANTICIPATIONS.

A WEEK LATER I WALKED OUT OF THE HILLS CARRYING WITHIN ME THE FAINTEST GLOW OF WHAT COULD HAVE BEEN **HOPE**. FOR THE FIRST TIME IN MONTHS MY VISION WASN'T BLURRED.

193

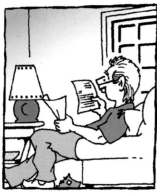

IN THE SAME WEEK, I RECEIVED TWO CRUCIAL COMMUNIQUÉS.

FOUR MONTHS AFTER MY ASSESSMENT, THE COUNSELLING SERVICE SENT ME AN APPOINTMENT FOR FRIDAY 16th MAY. IT DIDN'T BODE WELL. FRIDAY WAS ACTUALLY THE 13th.

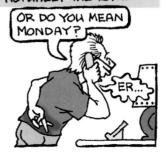

OR DO YOU MEAN MONDAY?

ER...

THEN THERE WAS THE LINE, 'LOW EARNERS ARE EXPECTED TO CONTRIBUTE £600 TOWARDS COSTS'.

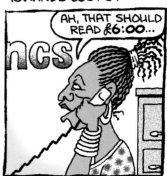

AH, THAT SHOULD READ £6:00...

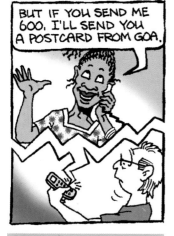

BUT IF YOU SEND ME 600, I'LL SEND YOU A POSTCARD FROM GOA.

THE SECOND WAS FROM THE CITY'S PSYCHOTHERAPY UNIT.

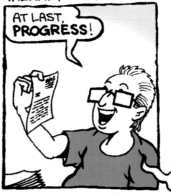

AT LAST, **PROGRESS!**

THREE MONTHS AFTER BEING REFERRED, THEY SENT ME A 12 PAGE QUESTIONAIRE WHICH, IF THEY LIKED MY ANSWERS, WOULD SPEED ME INTO AN INTERVIEW TWO MONTHS LATER WHICH, IF THEY LIKED MY ANSWERS, WOULD CATAPULT ME ONTO A WAITING LIST WHICH, IF EVERYTHING WENT ACCORDING TO THE LETTER, WOULD FAST-TRACK ME ONTO A THERAPIST'S COUCH **TWO YEARS** AFTER THAT.

WHOA, FEEL THE G-FORCE!

JUDY HAD WARNED ME...

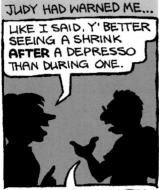

LIKE I SAID, Y'BETTER SEEING A SHRINK **AFTER** A DEPRESSO THAN DURING ONE.

BUT I'LL BE **FOUR YEARS** OLDER THAN WHEN I WAS FIRST DIAGNOSED...

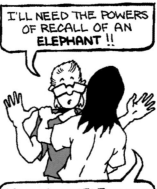

I'LL NEED THE POWERS OF RECALL OF AN **ELEPHANT** !!

CALM YOURSELF, SWEET PRINCE, YOU **WILL** EMERGE INTO THE LIGHT.

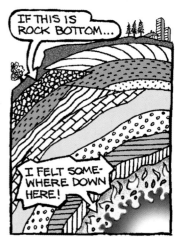

IF THIS IS ROCK BOTTOM...

I FELT SOMEWHERE DOWN HERE!

MEANTIME, OTHER WHEELS WERE TURNING. AS HARD AS I WAS TRYING TO JIMMY MY WAY INTO THE MENTAL HEALTH SYSTEM, THE BENEFITS SYSTEM WAS TRYING TO JIMMY ME OUT.

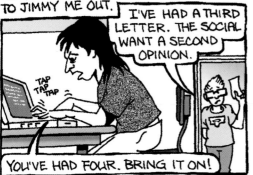

I'VE HAD A THIRD LETTER. THE SOCIAL WANT A SECOND OPINION.

TAP TAP TAP

YOU'VE HAD FOUR. BRING IT ON!

UNABLE TO WORK SINCE OUR RETURN FROM CHINA, I HAD BEEN RECEIVING £60 A WEEK INCAPACITY BENEFIT.

BUT I DON'T ACTUALLY FEEL ILL!

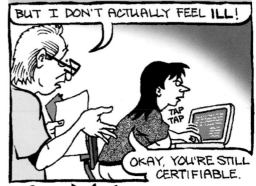

TAP TAP

OKAY, YOU'RE STILL CERTIFIABLE.

NOT THAT I WASN'T GRATEFUL, BUT I WAS NOW LIVING ON LESS THAN I COULD EARN FOR ONE CARTOON.

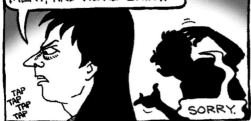

AS LONG AS I'VE KNOW YOU, YOU'VE WORKED YOU'RE PINKIES TO THE BONE TO BRING HOME THE BACON. SUDDENLY YOU'RE NEITHER USE NOR ORNAMENT, AND WE'RE SKINT.

TAP TAP TAP TAP

SORRY.

FUCK SORRY!! THAT'S ILL! YOU DON'T HAVE TO BE RAJ PERSAUD TO REALISE YOU'VE ATROPHIED.

ATRO-WHAT?

I DUNNO, TOM. I THOUGHT THE MOVE WOULD BE A FRESH START. LEAVE THE MISERY BEHIND. BUT YOU'RE TEARING ME APART HERE.

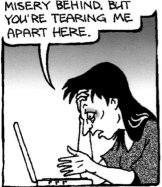

I'M NOT SURE I CAN COPE MUCH LONGER. FUCK'S SAKE, I WANT TO BE HAPPY!

I'M SORRY. YOU'VE ENOUGH ON YOUR PLATE.

I'M TRYING MY DAMNEDEST.

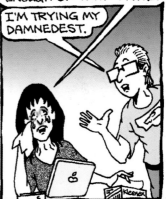

I HADN'T GIVEN THE FIRST THOUGHT TO THE TOLL MY BREAKDOWN WAS TAKING OF THOSE CLOSE TO ME.

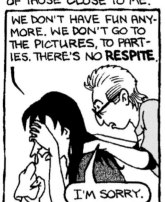

WE DON'T HAVE FUN ANYMORE. WE DON'T GO TO THE PICTURES, TO PARTIES. THERE'S NO **RESPITE**.

I'M SORRY.

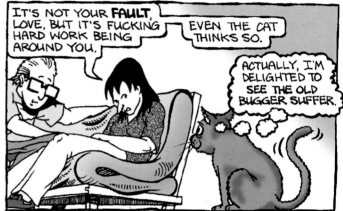

IT'S NOT YOUR **FAULT**, LOVE, BUT IT'S FUCKING HARD WORK BEING AROUND YOU.

EVEN THE CAT THINKS SO.

ACTUALLY, I'M DELIGHTED TO SEE THE OLD **BUGGER** SUFFER.

I HAD BECOME THE MOST SELFISH BASTARD IMAGINABLE. JUDY COULD HAVE BEEN **DYING** OF CANCER FOR ALL I CARED.

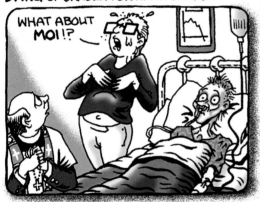

WHAT ABOUT **MOI**!?

NOTHING IN THE WORLD MATTERED MORE THAN ME, MOSTLY BECAUSE I HAD VANISHED WITHOUT TRACE. I WAS **MYOPIC** ABOUT FINDING ME, AND FAST, BEFORE SOMETHING REALLY FREAKY MOVED IN.

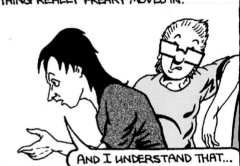

AND I UNDERSTAND THAT...

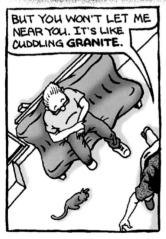

BUT YOU WON'T LET ME NEAR YOU. IT'S LIKE CUDDLING **GRANITE**.

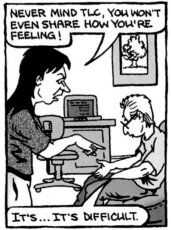

NEVER MIND TLC, YOU WON'T EVEN SHARE HOW YOU'RE FEELING!

IT'S... IT'S DIFFICULT.

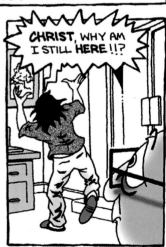

CHRIST, WHY AM I STILL **HERE**!!?

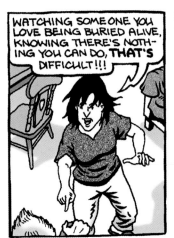

WATCHING SOMEONE YOU LOVE BEING BURIED ALIVE, KNOWING THERE'S NOTHING YOU CAN DO, **THAT'S** DIFFICULT!!!

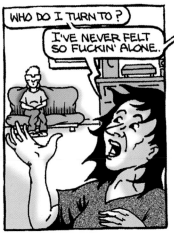

WHO DO I TURN TO?

I'VE NEVER FELT SO FUCKIN' ALONE.

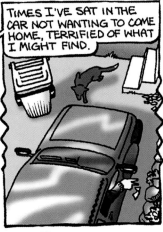

TIMES I'VE SAT IN THE CAR NOT WANTING TO COME HOME, TERRIFIED OF WHAT I MIGHT FIND.

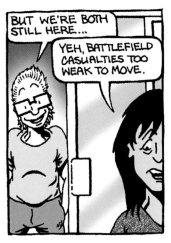

BUT WE'RE BOTH STILL HERE...

YEH, BATTLEFIELD CASUALTIES TOO WEAK TO MOVE.

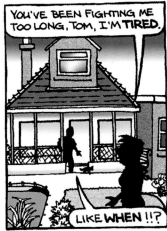

YOU'VE BEEN FIGHTING ME TOO LONG, TOM, I'M **TIRED.**

LIKE **WHEN** !!?

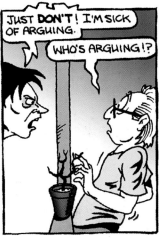

JUST **DON'T**! I'M SICK OF ARGUING.

WHO'S ARGUING!?

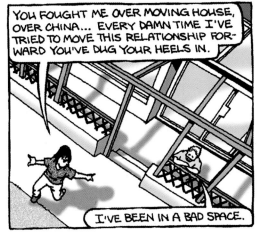

YOU FOUGHT ME OVER MOVING HOUSE, OVER CHINA... EVERY DAMN TIME I'VE TRIED TO MOVE THIS RELATIONSHIP FORWARD YOU'VE DUG YOUR HEELS IN.

I'VE BEEN IN A BAD SPACE.

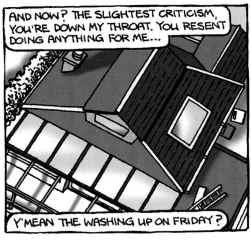

AND NOW? THE SLIGHTEST CRITICISM, YOU'RE DOWN MY THROAT. YOU RESENT DOING ANYTHING FOR ME...

Y'MEAN THE WASHING UP ON FRIDAY?

197

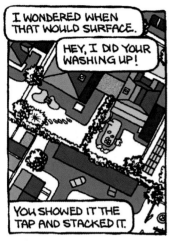

I WONDERED WHEN THAT WOULD SURFACE.

HEY, I DID YOUR WASHING UP!

YOU SHOWED IT THE TAP AND STACKED IT.

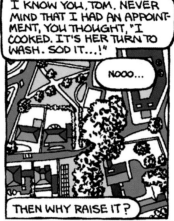

I KNOW YOU, TOM. NEVER MIND THAT I HAD AN APPOINTMENT, YOU THOUGHT, "I COOKED. IT'S HER TURN TO WASH. SOD IT...!"

NOOO...

THEN WHY RAISE IT?

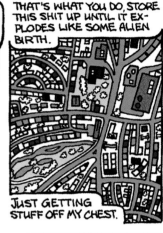

THAT'S WHAT YOU DO, STORE THIS SHIT UP UNTIL IT EXPLODES LIKE SOME ALIEN BIRTH.

JUST GETTING STUFF OFF MY CHEST.

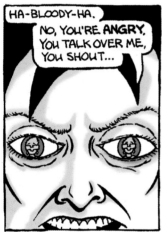

HA-BLOODY-HA.

NO, YOU'RE **ANGRY**, YOU TALK OVER ME, YOU SHOUT...

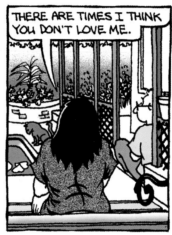

THERE ARE TIMES I THINK YOU DON'T LOVE ME.

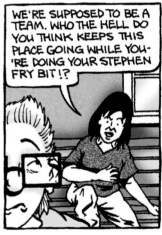

WE'RE SUPPOSED TO BE A TEAM. WHO THE HELL DO YOU THINK KEEPS THIS PLACE GOING WHILE YOU'RE DOING YOUR STEPHEN FRY BIT!?

PROBABLY I DID HOLD BACK. I WAS SUCH A STRONG SILENT STEREOTYPE I EMBARRASSED MYSELF.

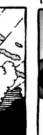

WHAT DID I UNDERSTAND ABOUT RELATIONSHIPS?

I DIDN'T KNOW ANY WOMEN UNTIL I WAS 18, A MOTHER INCLUDED. DIDN'T SEE ONE NAKED UNTIL I WAS 24!

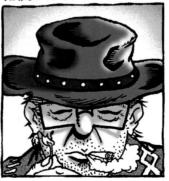

MY CLOSEST BUDDIES—THE ONES I CAN REALLY TALK TO—HAVE SINCE BEEN WOMEN.

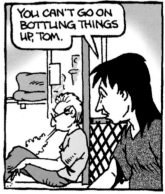

YOU CAN'T GO ON BOTTLING THINGS UP, TOM.

BUT I FELL IN LOVE WITH JUDY WITHOUT PASSING THROUGH FRIENDSHIP.

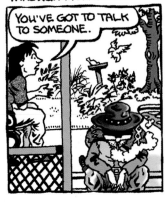

YOU'VE GOT TO TALK TO SOMEONE.

THE YEARS STRIPPED AWAY THE ARMOUR, BUT THE CLOSER WE GOT THE MORE DIFFICULT IT BECAME FOR ME.

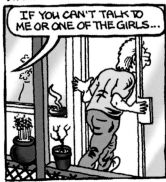

IF YOU CAN'T TALK TO ME OR ONE OF THE GIRLS...

YES I HELD BACK, HORDING MY DEEPEST INSECURITIES, CONVINCED JUDY WOULD WALK AWAY SOME DAY.

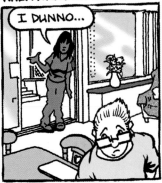

I DUNNO...

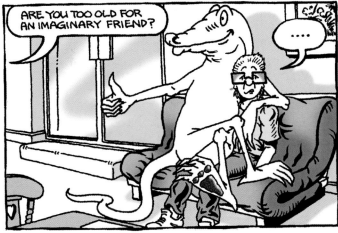

ARE YOU TOO OLD FOR AN IMAGINARY FRIEND?

....

ONE MORTAL WOUNDING IS ENOUGH IN A LIFETIME.

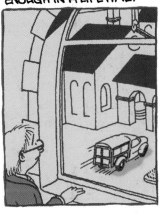

THEN SOMETHING **EXTRAORDINARY** HAPPENED. OUT OF THE STAGNANT DARKNESS A HELPING HAND APPEARED. IN FACT **TWO**.

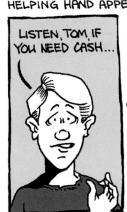

LISTEN, TOM, IF YOU NEED CASH...

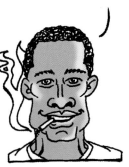

DON'T BE TOO PROUD TO ASK...

OR ANY KIND OF HELP...

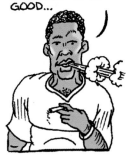

LIKE WE KNOW THIS RETIRED PSYCHOTHERAPIST, 'SUPPOSED TO BE GOOD...

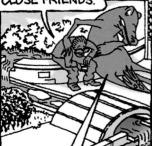

I WAS **CHOKED**. THEY WEREN'T PARTICULARLY CLOSE FRIENDS.

DON'T EXPECT TO HAVE THE SAME FRIENDS IN HELL YOU HAD IN PURGATORY.

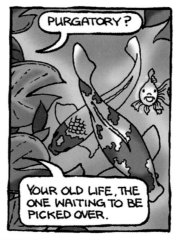

PURGATORY?

YOUR OLD LIFE, THE ONE WAITING TO BE PICKED OVER.

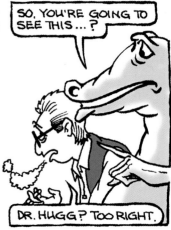

SO, YOU'RE GOING TO SEE THIS...?

DR. HUGG? TOO RIGHT.

FIVE YEARS AGO, IF ANYBODY HAD SAID A DAY WOULD COME WHEN I'D BE JUMPING FOR JOY ABOUT GOING TO SEE A SHRINK...

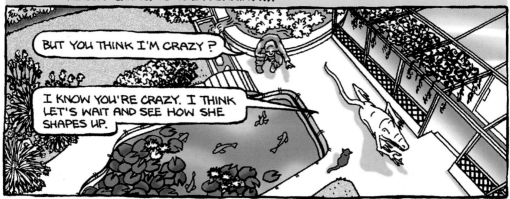

BUT YOU THINK I'M CRAZY?

I KNOW YOU'RE CRAZY. I THINK LET'S WAIT AND SEE HOW SHE SHAPES UP.

HUGG LIVED AN HOUR'S RIDE AWAY, WITH ENOUGH HILLS BETWEEN US TO ENSURE I GOT SOMETHING OUT OF A VISIT, IF ONLY AN ENDORPHIN RUSH.

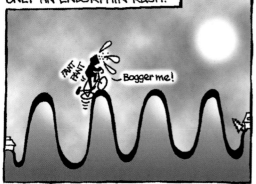

PANT PANT

Bogger me!

SHE HAD RETIRED FROM A BIG MONEY GAME, WHICH MEANT POSH HOUSE, FLASH CAR, CHARGE ACCOUNTS, DIFFERENT PLANET, BUT HEY, SUCK IT AND...

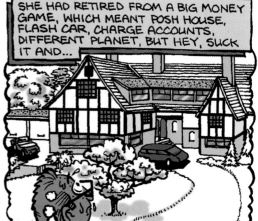

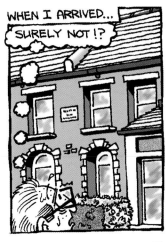

WHEN I ARRIVED... SURELY NOT!?

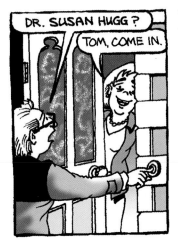

DR. SUSAN HUGG?

TOM, COME IN.

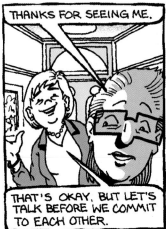

THANKS FOR SEEING ME.

THAT'S OKAY, BUT LET'S TALK BEFORE WE COMMIT TO EACH OTHER.

TELL ME SOME OF YOUR STORY, TOM.

WELL...

AS I SKIMMED THROUGH THE PAST COUPLE OF **ANNI HORRIBILIS**, I SCRUTINIZED HER SITTING ROOM.

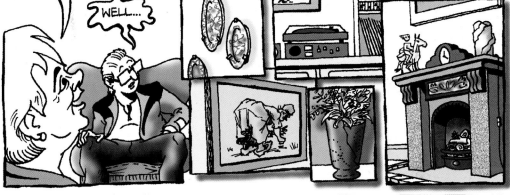

HUGG HAD TASTE. NOT A WHIFF OF **IKEA**!

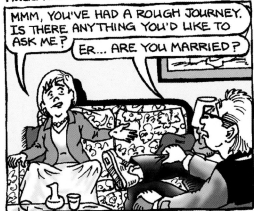

MMM, YOU'VE HAD A ROUGH JOURNEY. IS THERE ANYTHING YOU'D LIKE TO ASK ME?

ER... ARE YOU MARRIED?

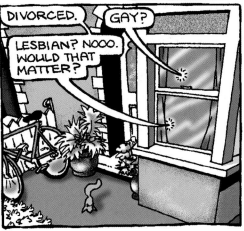

DIVORCED.

GAY?

LESBIAN? NOOO. WOULD THAT MATTER?

201

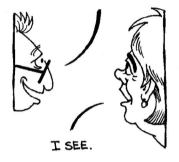

WELL, I GUESS WE'LL BE GETTING DEEP DOWN AND DIRTY. WOULDN'T WANT TO BE AMBUSHED BY YOUR INNER **MANEATER.**

I SEE.

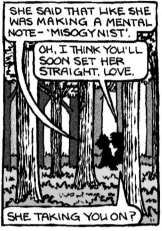

SHE SAID THAT LIKE SHE WAS MAKING A MENTAL NOTE - 'MISOGYNIST'.

OH, I THINK YOU'LL SOON SET HER STRAIGHT, LOVE.

SHE TAKING YOU ON?

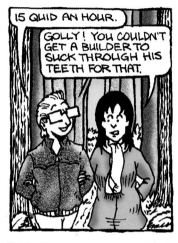

15 QUID AN HOUR.

GOLLY! YOU COULDN'T GET A BUILDER TO SUCK THROUGH HIS TEETH FOR THAT.

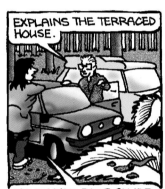

EXPLAINS THE TERRACED HOUSE.

MAYBE YOU POSE AN IRRESISTIBLE CHALLENGE? WHATEVER, YOU'RE ON YOUR WAY...

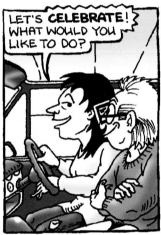

LET'S **CELEBRATE!** WHAT WOULD YOU LIKE TO DO?

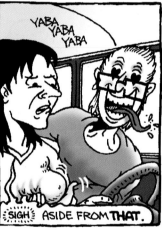

YABA YABA YABA

SIGH ASIDE FROM **THAT.**

MY FAVOURITE MUSICAL WAS PLAYING THE BIG SCREEN, COLOUR RESTORED WITH DIGITALLY ENHANCED SOUND.

DO DALOO DO
DO DA
DO DALOO DOO

DEEP IN THE VACUUM, I FELT A FLICKER OF OPTIMISM AND HUMMED ALONG.

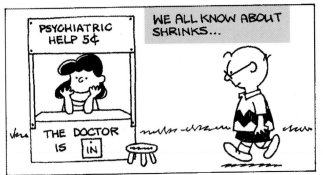

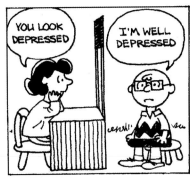

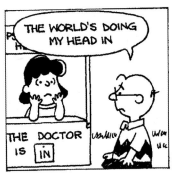

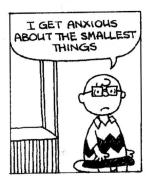

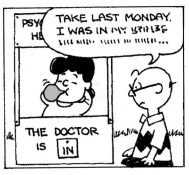

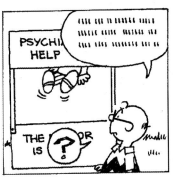

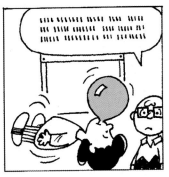

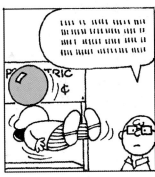

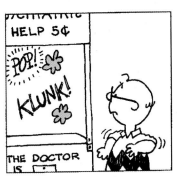

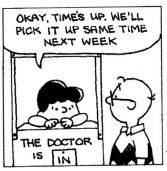

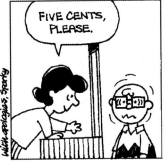

203

WE KNOW ABOUT FREUD AND HIS COUCH, AMERICANS AND THEIR ANALYSTS, CARTOONISTS AND THEIR DAFT JOKES...

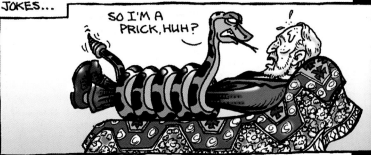

SO I'M A PRICK, HUH?

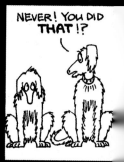

NEVER! YOU DID **THAT**!?

Receptio

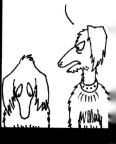

YOU NEED TO SEE A SHRINK, PAL.

AND WE KNOW ABOUT PAYING THROUGH THE NOSE FOR ANSWERS YOUR WIFE OR PARTNER WILL GIVE YOU FOR **FREE**.

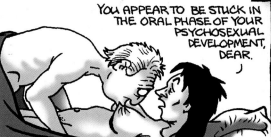

YOU APPEAR TO BE STUCK IN THE ORAL PHASE OF YOUR PSYCHOSEXUAL DEVELOPMENT, DEAR.

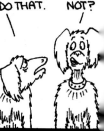

OH, I COULDN'T DO THAT.

AND WHY NOT?

BUT FOR AS LONG AS THERE HAS BEEN NOWT SO QUEER AS FOLK, SOCIETIES PRIMITIVE AND OTHERWISE HAVE HAD THEIR SHRINKS; STRANGERS WHO MIGHT HAVE INSIGHT INTO WHAT WE CAN'T SEE FOR LOOKING.

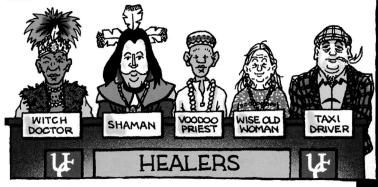

WITCH DOCTOR — SHAMAN — VOODOO PRIEST — WISE OLD WOMAN — TAXI DRIVER

HEALERS

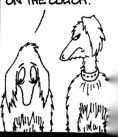

I'M NOT ALLOWED ON THE COUCH.

IT WAS GOOD TALKING TO HUGG. I LIKED HER. WE HAD A SIMILAR WORLD VIEW.

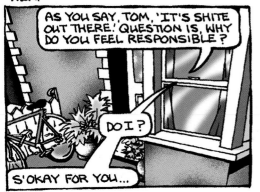

AS YOU SAY, TOM, 'IT'S SHITE OUT THERE!' QUESTION IS, WHY DO YOU FEEL RESPONSIBLE?

DO I?

S'OKAY FOR YOU...

WORSE IT GETS, LONGER THE QUEUE AT YOUR DOOR.

AND WHY SO BITTER?

NEEDLESS TO SAY I SPENT A MONTH OF TUESDAYS BEATING ABOUT THE BUSH, WHINGEING ABOUT THE THORNS.

THEN, ONE VISIT, I SAID SOMETHING THEN SHE SAID SOMETHING THEN I SAID, 'OH MA GAWD!' AND A FLOOD GATE OPENED – JUST A LITTLE ONE, MORE A SLUICE-GATE.

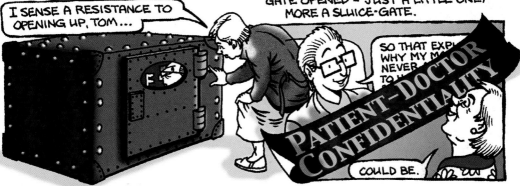

I SENSE A RESISTANCE TO OPENING UP, TOM...

SO THAT EXPL[...] WHY MY M[...] NEVER [...] TO H[...]

PATIENT-DOCTOR CONFIDENTIALITY

COULD BE.

MOST SESSIONS WERE LIKE...

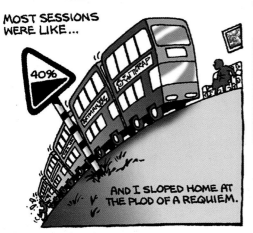

40%

AND I SLOPED HOME AT THE PLOD OF A REQUIEM.

BUT INCREASINGLY LITTLE REVELATIONS SHED LIGHT ON CORNERS OF THE DUNGEON I HAD APPARENTLY BUILT FOR MYSELF.

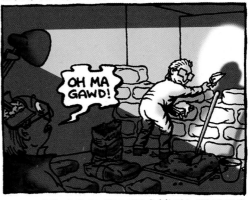

OH MA GAWD!

I RODE AWAY ON A HIGH, TAPPING A DANCE BEAT ON THE PEDALS.

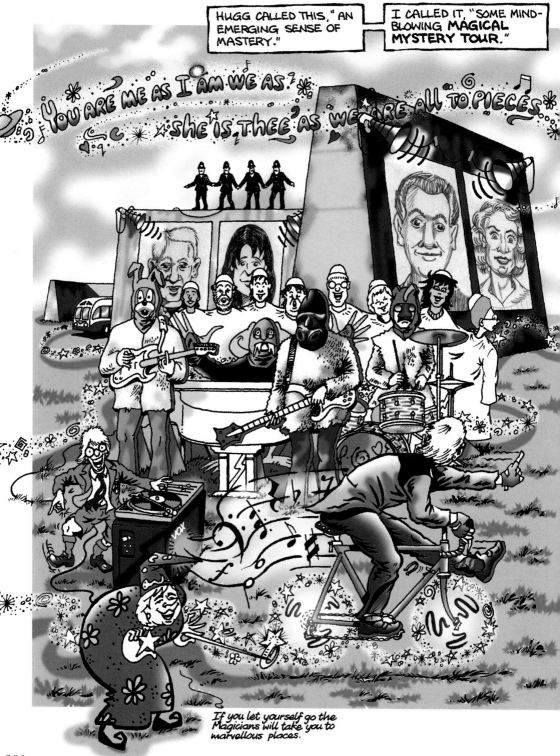

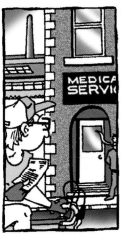

A MONTH INTO THERAPY I WAS SUMMONED BY THE BUNCH WHO SNIFF OUT SICKY-PULLERS FOR THE BENEFITS OFFICE.

WELCOME TO MEDICAL SERVICES
ZERO TOLERANCE
NO...
SHOUTING
SWEARING
FIGHTING
LYNCHINGS
SHOOT-OUTS

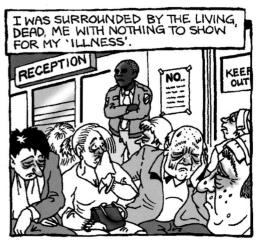

I WAS SURROUNDED BY THE LIVING DEAD, ME WITH NOTHING TO SHOW FOR MY 'ILLNESS'.

RECEPTION

NO.

KEEP OUT

WORSE. WITH ALL THE BACK AND FORTH TO HUGG'S, I STOOD OUT AS A PICTURE OF HEALTH.

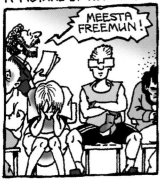

MEESTA FREEMUN!

THE SECOND OPINION WAS TO BE PROVIDED BY A GREEK DOCTOR WHOSE ENGLISH WAS AS FLUENT AS MY GREEK.

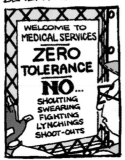

Πᾶσα τέχνη καὶ πᾶσα μέθοδος, ὁμοίως δὲ πρᾶξίς τε καὶ προαίρεσις.

THE ILIAD, RIGHT?

IT RESTED ON MY ANSWERS TO INCISIVE QUESTIONS LIKE, "CAN YOU USE A VACUUM CLEANER?"...

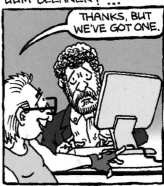

THANKS, BUT WE'VE GOT ONE.

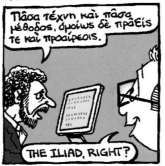

AND...

NO...

F'SURE I TIDY UP AFTER MYSELF. I'VE A WIFE!!

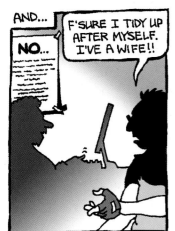

I LEFT CONVINCED HE WOULD PASS ME FIT FOR A **BRILLIANT NEW CAREER.**

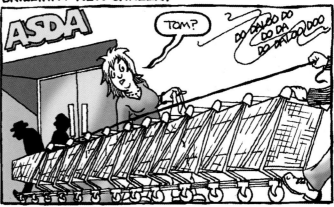

ASDA

TOM?

DO DADOO DO DO DA DO DADOO DOO

(PERVERSELY, I QUITE FANCIED BEING SHOED INTO **GRUNT WORK** FOR SOME WANKY YANKIE MULTINATIONAL, I WAS DIAGNOSED BONKERS, A FAILSAFE EXCUSE FOR FUN FUN **FUN!**)

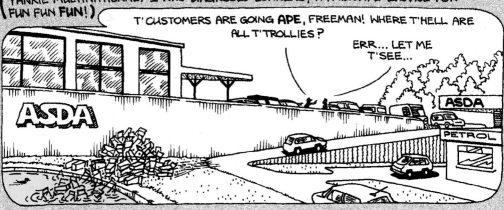

T'CUSTOMERS ARE GOING **APE**, FREEMAN! WHERE T'HELL ARE ALL T'TROLLIES?

ERR... LET ME T'SEE...

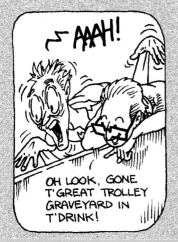

~AAAH!

OH LOOK, GONE T'GREAT TROLLEY GRAVEYARD IN T'DRINK!

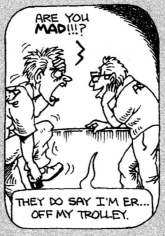

ARE YOU **MAD!!!?**

THEY DO SAY I'M ER... OFF MY TROLLEY.

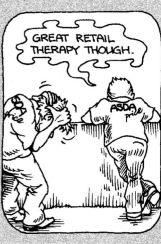

GREAT RETAIL THERAPY THOUGH.

THE CLOCK IN THE JOB CENTRE WAS NOW COUNTING DOWN. IN THE HOPE THAT **TWO** THERAPISTS WOULD BE MORE PRODUCTIVE THAN ONE, I KEPT MY APPOINTMENT WITH N.C.S.

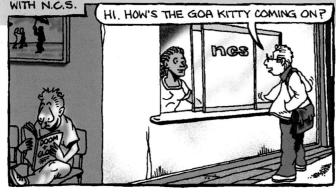

HI. HOW'S THE GOA KITTY COMING ON?

COMPARED TO HUGG'S PLACE, THE DECOR WAS CAR BOOT.

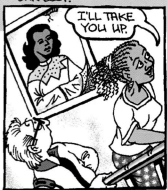

I'LL TAKE YOU UP.

IT GOT MORE RECYCLED THE HIGHER WE CLIMBED.

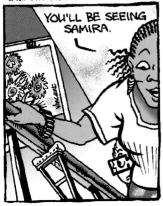

YOU'LL BE SEEING SAMIRA.

OUR ROOM WAS IN THE ATTIC.

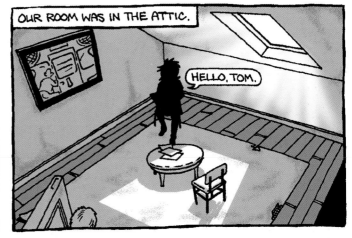

HELLO, TOM.

THE ONLY PICTURE WAS A FADED WOOLWORTH PRINT, POPULAR IN 1960'S KARDOHMAS.

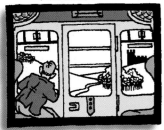

I SPENT MOST OF THE SESSION WILLING THE TRAIN TO MOVE.

THE PROBLEM WAS SAM-IRA. SHE WAS A TANNED, TOP-HEAVY VERSION OF JUDY TEN YEARS AGO...

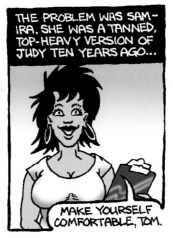

MAKE YOURSELF COMFORTABLE, TOM.

COMPELLINGLY TOP-HEAVY!!

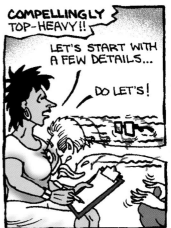

LET'S START WITH A FEW DETAILS...

DO LET'S!

I SHUDDER TO THINK WHAT MIGHT HAVE **BEFALLEN** THE POOR GIRL WERE IT NOT FOR THAT PICTURE.

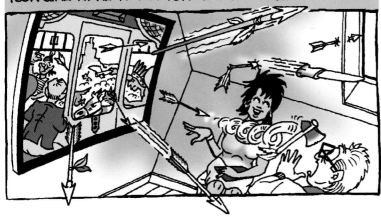

IT WAS THE SCARIEST HOUR OF MY LIFE.

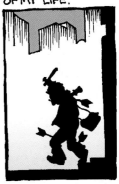

I DIDN'T GO BACK.

209

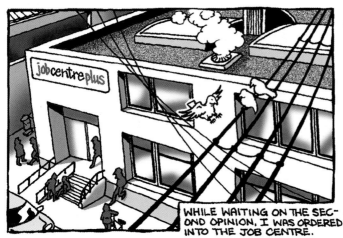

THE **PLUS** IS THEIR WAY OF REMINDING US THAT THE BENEFITS COMPUTER IS LINKED TO THE EMPLOYMENT, HEALTH, REVENUE, IMMIGRATION, POLICE, COUNTER INTELLIGENCE AND PROBABLY YOUR WASHING MACHINE'S COMPUTER.

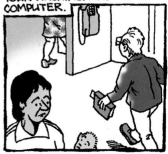

WHILE WAITING ON THE SECOND OPINION, I WAS ORDERED INTO THE JOB CENTRE.

(THERE ARE **72** INTERFACES IN WHITEHALL'S COMPUTER INTELLIGENCE WEB, AN APPARATUS OF CONTROL SECOND ONLY TO CHINA'S 'GOLD SHIELD PROJECT'.

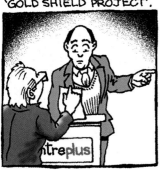

THIS MEANS EITHER A) YOU CAN'T TAKE A CRAP WITHOUT THEM KNOWING WHEN, WHERE AND WHAT CONSISTENCY OR ...

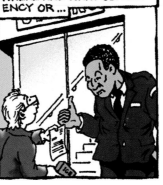

B) YOUR RECORDS HAVE VANISHED, NOW IN THE HANDS OF I.D. FRAUDSTERS.)

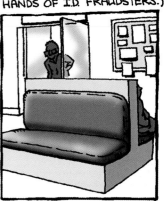

GOOD READ?

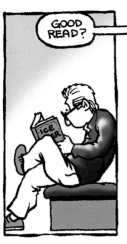

GARETH, HI. I'M YOUR SPECIALIST INCAPACITY ADVISER.

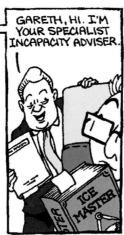

NOTHING TO WORRY ABOUT, TOM. JUST TO BRING YOU UP TO SPEED WITH WHAT WE CAN DO FOR YOU.

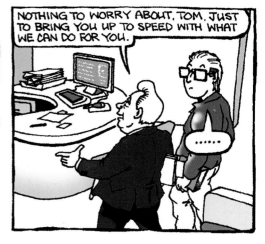

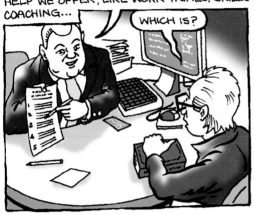

THIS IS A LIST OF FINANCIAL AND CAREERS HELP WE OFFER, LIKE WORK TRIALS, SKILLS COACHING...

WHICH IS?

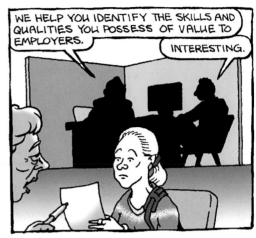

WE HELP YOU IDENTIFY THE SKILLS AND QUALITIES YOU POSSESS OF VALUE TO EMPLOYERS.

INTERESTING.

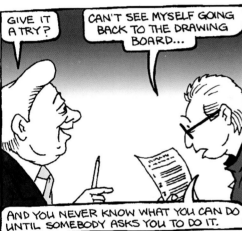

GIVE IT A TRY?

CAN'T SEE MYSELF GOING BACK TO THE DRAWING BOARD...

AND YOU NEVER KNOW WHAT YOU CAN DO UNTIL SOMEBODY ASKS YOU TO DO IT.

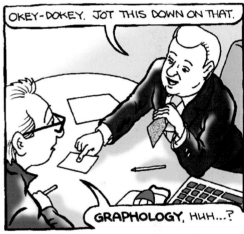

OKEY-DOKEY. JOT THIS DOWN ON THAT.

GRAPHOLOGY, HUH...?

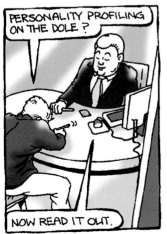

PERSONALITY PROFILING ON THE DOLE?

NOW READ IT OUT.

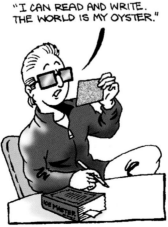

"I CAN READ AND WRITE. THE WORLD IS MY OYSTER."

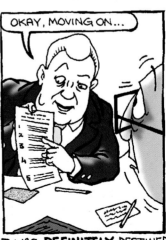

OKAY, MOVING ON...

I WAS **DEFINITELY** DESTINED FOR ASDA'S FORECOURT.

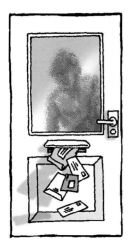

A COUPLE OF WEEKS LATER, GARETH INFORMED ME I WOULDN'T NEED TO PROVIDE ANOTHER SICK NOTE FOR **18 MONTHS**!

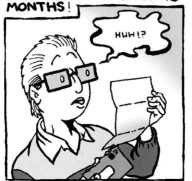

HUH!?

THE SECOND OPINION WAS IN. THEY WERE LIFTING THE PRESSURE ON ME TO FIND WORK.

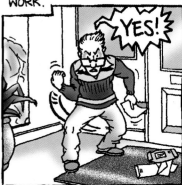

YES!

MY RELIEF WAS...

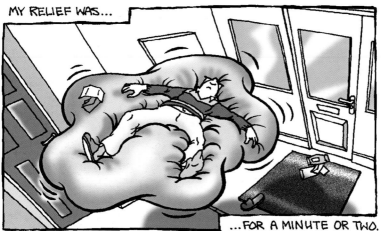

...FOR A MINUTE OR TWO.

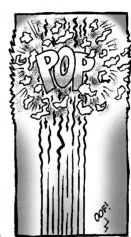

POP

OOF!

18 MONTHS HASSLE-FREE BENEFITS? **THIS** GOVERNMENT!?

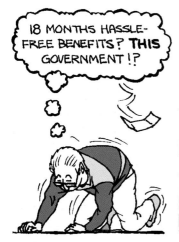

WHAT DID THE **GEEKY GREEK** FIND? WHAT LURKING PSYCHOSIS WAS UNMASKED BY HIS DEVILISH INTERROGATION?

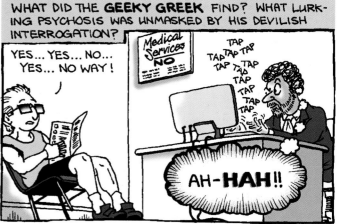

YES... YES... NO... YES... NO WAY!

Medical Services NO

TAP TAP TAP TAP TAP TAP TAP TAP TAP TAP TAP TAP

AH-**HAH**!!

WERE MULTIPLE PERSONALITIES POISED FOR A MASS BREAK-OUT ...

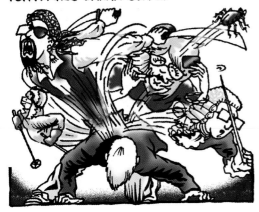

WOULD I SPROUT WHISKERS AND FANGS AT THE NEXT FULL MOON ...

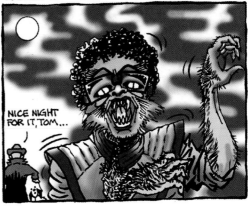

NICE NIGHT FOR IT, TOM ...

AND WHY WASN'T HUGG REMOTELY CONCERNED?

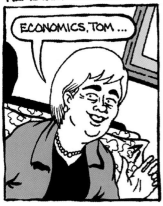

ECONOMICS, TOM ...

YOU'RE WORTH MORE TO THE TAXMAN AS A CARTOONIST THAN AS A BRICKY'S MATE.

I WASN'T SHOOTING THAT HIGH...

AH, YES, YOUR SHOPPING TROLLEY DREAMS...

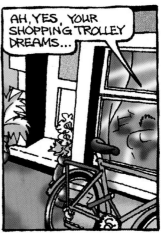

WITHOUT A DOUBT I WAS A DEPRESSO, BUT OF WHAT ORDER? WAS I **CLINICAL** WITH A SIDE ORDER OF **ANXIETY NEUROSIS**, OR MAY BE **DYSTHYMIC**, MARINATED IN A RICH **DYSPHORIC** SAUCE?

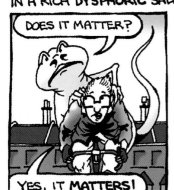

DOES IT MATTER?

YES, IT MATTERS!

IF I KNOW WHAT I AM...

WHAT, YOU CAN FIX IT!? YOU'VE SAID NO TO DRUGS, WHAT'S TO KNOW?

AND WHAT IS DYSTHYMICY-BOB!!?

I'D LOOK IT UP.

SURE, WHY NOT ADD TO YOUR CONFUSION?

213

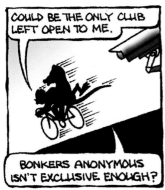

COULD BE THE ONLY CLUB LEFT OPEN TO ME.

BONKERS ANONYMOUS ISN'T EXCLUSIVE ENOUGH?

MAYBE I WAS JUST LONELY, BUT I SUDDENLY FELT THE NEED TO MEET OTHER CRAZIES.

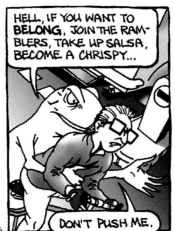

HELL, IF YOU WANT TO **BELONG**, JOIN THE RAMBLERS, TAKE UP SALSA, BECOME A CHRISPY...

DON'T PUSH ME.

PERHAPS I THOUGHT SHARING MISERIES WOULD BE REASSURING, EVEN **UPLIFTING** IF I COULD FIND A BUNCH OF WACKOS THAT MADE ME LOOK SANE.

IT IS EASY FOR A DEPRESSO TO DISTINGUISH A FELLOW TRAVELLER FROM THE MASS OF MISERABLE BUGGERS HAVING AN AVERAGE DAY. IT'S THE DEAD EYES AND CRYOGENIC FEATURES.

I GOT TALKING TO NAZ OUTSIDE THE SURGERY...

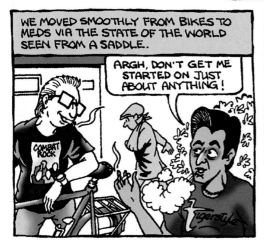

WE MOVED SMOOTHLY FROM BIKES TO MEDS VIA THE STATE OF THE WORLD SEEN FROM A SADDLE.

ARGH, DON'T GET ME STARTED ON JUST ABOUT ANYTHING!

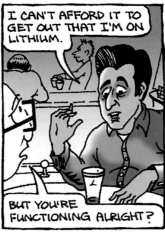

WE MET A COUPLE OF TIMES FOR A BEER AND SWAPPED RIPPING YARNS OF DAILY DESPAIR, BAFFLED QUACKS AND LIFE ON THE SMARTIES.

I WORK IN THE NHS. PRACTISE MANAGER AT BEESTON CLINIC.

THAT'LL DO IT...

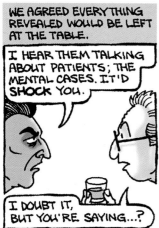

WE AGREED EVERYTHING REVEALED WOULD BE LEFT AT THE TABLE.

I HEAR THEM TALKING ABOUT PATIENTS; THE MENTAL CASES. IT'D **SHOCK** YOU.

I DOUBT IT, BUT YOU'RE SAYING...?

I CAN'T AFFORD IT TO GET OUT THAT I'M ON LITHIUM.

BUT YOU'RE FUNCTIONING ALRIGHT?

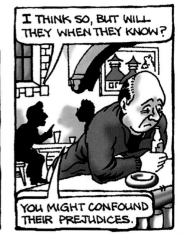

I THINK SO, BUT WILL THEY WHEN THEY KNOW?

YOU MIGHT CONFOUND THEIR PREJUDICES.

214

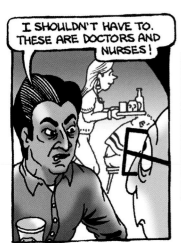

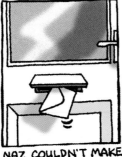

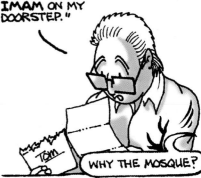

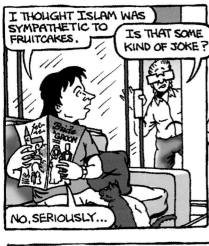

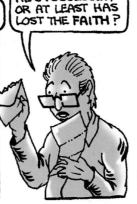

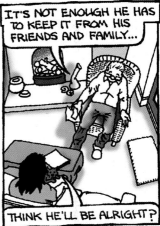

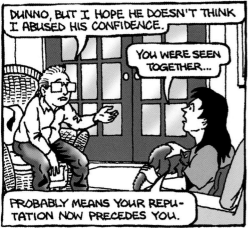

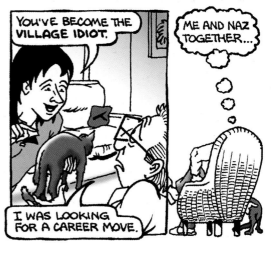

215

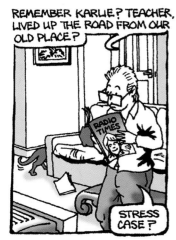

REMEMBER KARLIE? TEACHER, LIVED UP THE ROAD FROM OUR OLD PLACE?

STRESS CASE?

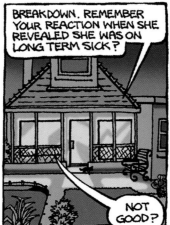

BREAKDOWN. REMEMBER YOUR REACTION WHEN SHE REVEALED SHE WAS ON LONG TERM SICK?

NOT GOOD?

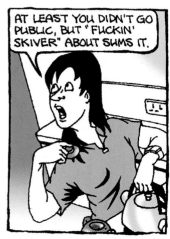

AT LEAST YOU DIDN'T GO PUBLIC, BUT "FUCKIN' SKIVER" ABOUT SUMS IT.

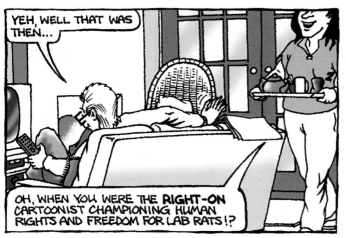

YEH, WELL THAT WAS THEN...

OH, WHEN YOU WERE THE **RIGHT-ON** CARTOONIST CHAMPIONING HUMAN RIGHTS AND FREEDOM FOR LAB RATS!?

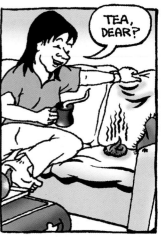

TEA, DEAR?

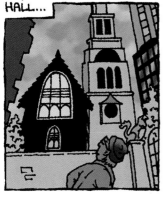

MY NEXT ATTEMPT TO MEET A KINDRED SPIRIT (OR LACK OF) TOOK ME TO A CHURCH HALL....

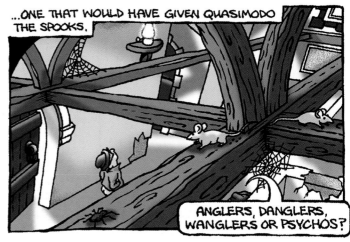

...ONE THAT WOULD HAVE GIVEN QUASIMODO THE SPOOKS.

ANGLERS, DANGLERS, WANGLERS OR PSYCHOS?

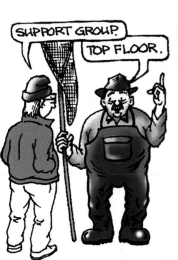

SUPPORT GROUP?

TOP FLOOR.

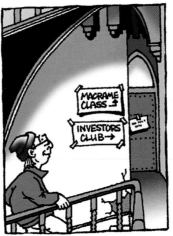

MACRAME CLASS →

INVESTORS CLUB →

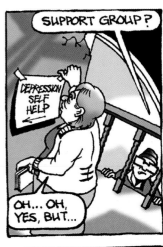

SUPPORT GROUP?

DEPRESSION SELF HELP ←

OH... OH, YES, BUT...

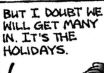

BUT I DOUBT WE WILL GET MANY IN. IT'S THE HOLIDAYS.

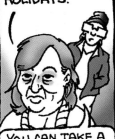

YOU CAN TAKE A HOLIDAY FROM DEPRESSION!?

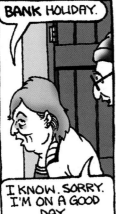

BANK HOLIDAY.

I KNOW. SORRY. I'M ON A GOOD DAY...

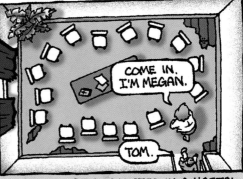

COME IN. I'M MEGAN.

TOM.

THE ROOM WAS DECORATED IN A NOSTAL-GIC COAT OF TOBACCO STAIN, BUT THE WILTING PLASTIC CHEESEPLANT IN THE CORNER WAS A HOMELY TOUCH.

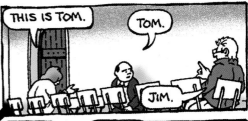

THIS IS TOM.

TOM.

JIM.

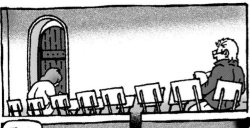

JIM.

MEGAN.

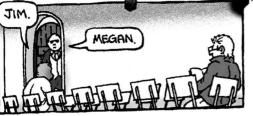

POLLY?

MEGAN?

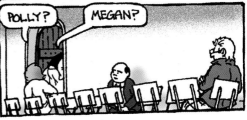

217

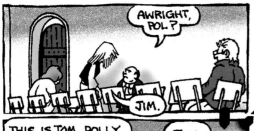

AWRIGHT, POL?

JIM.

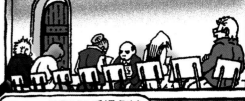

... AND SO ON UNTIL THERE WERE SIX OF US.

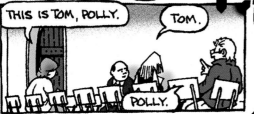

THIS IS TOM, POLLY.

TOM.

POLLY.

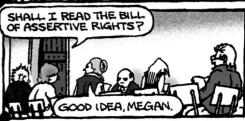

SHALL I READ THE BILL OF ASSERTIVE RIGHTS?

GOOD IDEA, MEGAN.

EVEN READ WITH ALL THE EXPRESSIVE TONALITY OF A DIRGE, THE BILL WAS GOOD STUFF.

You have the right to make mistakes and be responsible for them.
You have the right to change your mind.
You have the right to say 'I don't know'.
You have the right to relate to people without liking them or being liked.
You have the right to choose what you care about.
You have the right to say NO without feeling guilty.

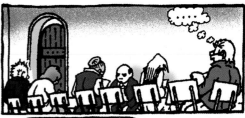

SHALL I START?

GOOD IDEA, POL.

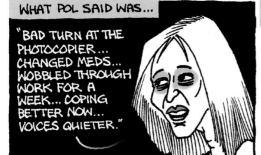

WHAT POL SAID WAS...

"BAD TURN AT THE PHOTOCOPIER... CHANGED MEDS... WOBBLED THROUGH WORK FOR A WEEK... COPING BETTER NOW... VOICES QUIETER."

... EXCEPT IT TOOK HALF AN HOUR, SOUNDED LIKE HER DEATH RATTLE AND SHE'D BEEN REPEATING THE CYCLE EVERY FEW MONTHS FOR SIX YEARS.

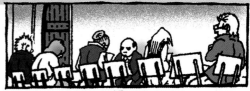

THEY WERE RUNNING OUT OF DRUGS TO TRY ON POL. SHE WAS A MESS.

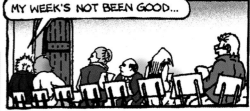

MY WEEK'S NOT BEEN GOOD...

THREE HOURS OF **TALES FROM UNDER THE CHEMICAL COSH** LEFT ME DRAINED. WHAT LITTLE HEART I HAD WENT OUT TO THE POOR BUGGERS.

WILL WE SEE YOU NEXT WEEK, TOM?

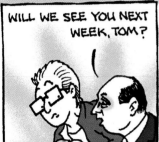

OKAY, **SOME DRUGS ARE USEFUL FOR SOME PEOPLE**, BUT C'MON...

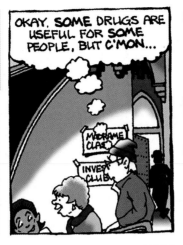

HOW MANY ZOMBIES ARE ARE THERE OUT HERE!?

ENOUGH FOR AN UPRISING?

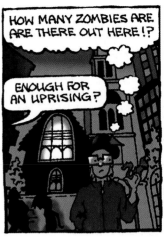

Y'THINK IT SMACKS OF **SOCIAL CONTROL?**

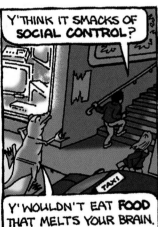

Y'WOULDN'T EAT **FOOD** THAT MELTS YOUR BRAIN.

WOULDN'T BE ON THE THE SHELVES.

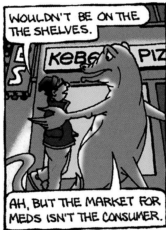

AH, BUT THE MARKET FOR MEDS ISN'T THE CONSUMER.

WE FORK OUT FOR THE DAMN THINGS!!

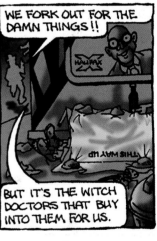

BUT IT'S THE WITCH DOCTORS THAT BUY INTO THEM FOR US.

FORGET **CONSUMER RIGHTS.** WE JUST TAKE WHAT WE'RE GIVEN, LIKE YOU DID.

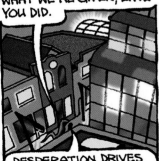

DESPERATION DRIVES FOLK TO IRRATIONAL PRACTISES, PAL...

BUT THE HELL I WENT THROUGH IN THE CAMBRIANS WAS A PICNIC BY COMPARISON WITH THAT SHIT.

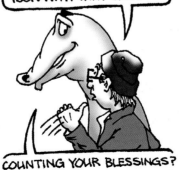

COUNTING YOUR BLESSINGS?

TOO RIGHT!

PRAISE THE LORD...

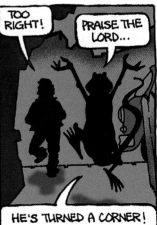

HE'S TURNED A CORNER!

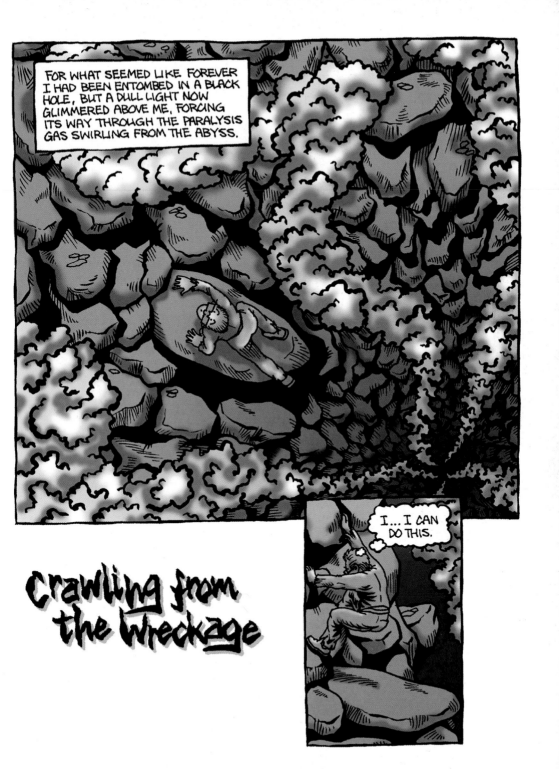

FOR WHAT SEEMED LIKE FOREVER I HAD BEEN ENTOMBED IN A BLACK HOLE, BUT A DULL LIGHT NOW GLIMMERED ABOVE ME, FORCING ITS WAY THROUGH THE PARALYSIS GAS SWIRLING FROM THE ABYSS.

Crawling from the Wreckage

I... I CAN DO THIS.

IT APPEARED I WAS CLIMBING, INITIALLY GAINING HEIGHT SURPRISINGLY SWIFTLY. BUT EACH DAY THE GRADIENT SLACKENED. THE ASCENT GOT EASIER BUT THE CONTOURS CONQUERED GOT LESS.

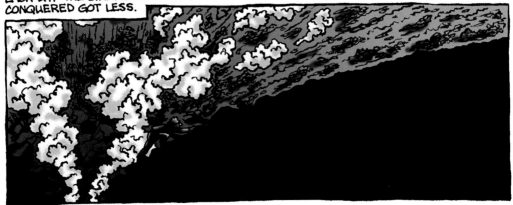

AND THE SURFACE BECAME LESS STABLE. WHERE ROCKS AND CREVASSES PROVIDED FIRM HOLDS AND LEVERS, RAMMEL AND SCREE NOW FRUSTRATED PROGRESS. I WAS UNLIKELY TO TUMBLE ALL THE WAY BACK, BUT WHO KNOWS WHAT LAY AHEAD.

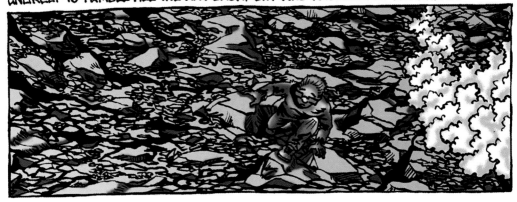

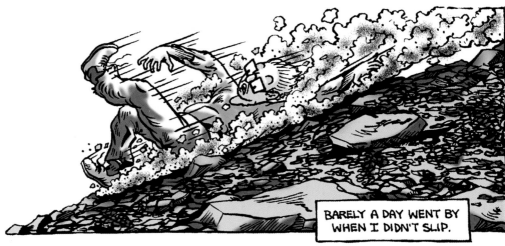

BARELY A DAY WENT BY WHEN I DIDN'T SLIP.

BUT I **WAS** FEELING BETTER.

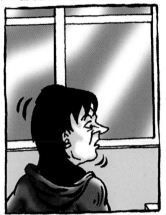

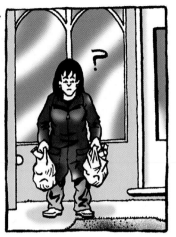

?

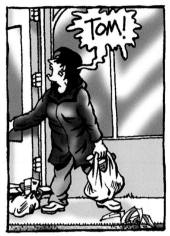

TOM!

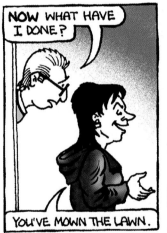

NOW WHAT HAVE I DONE?

YOU'VE MOWN THE LAWN.

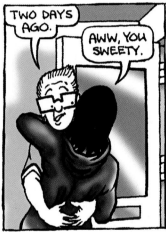

TWO DAYS AGO.

AWW, YOU SWEETY.

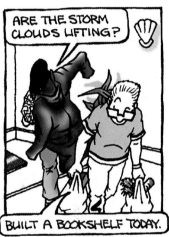

ARE THE STORM CLOUDS LIFTING?

BUILT A BOOKSHELF TODAY.

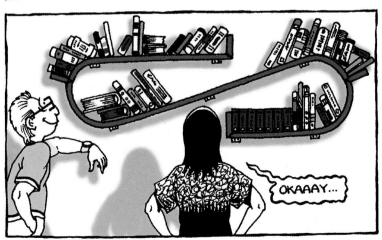

OKAAAY...

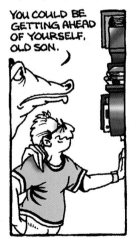

YOU COULD BE GETTING AHEAD OF YOURSELF, OLD SON.

223

THE TIDE WAS BEGINNING TO **TURN**. I WAS PHYSICALLY ACTIVE, IN THERAPY, GRANTED TIME, AND LEARNING TO COPE ON A PAUPER'S MITE.

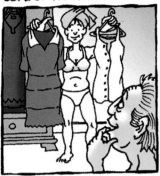

THERE WERE MOMENTS OF JOLITY WITH JUDY. WAVES OF NEW-FOUND LOVE FLOWED BETWEEN US.

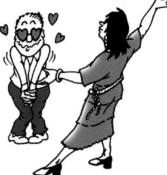

WE EVEN DID A PARTY **TOGETHER**, WHICH TOOK COURAGE. THE HOST WAS OUR YOGA TEACHER.

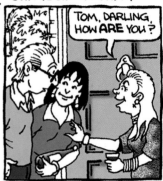

TOM, DARLING, HOW **ARE** YOU?

FOR A FULL FRIGHTENING HOUR I WAS TRAPPED IN A **POSY SIMMONDS** CARTOON.

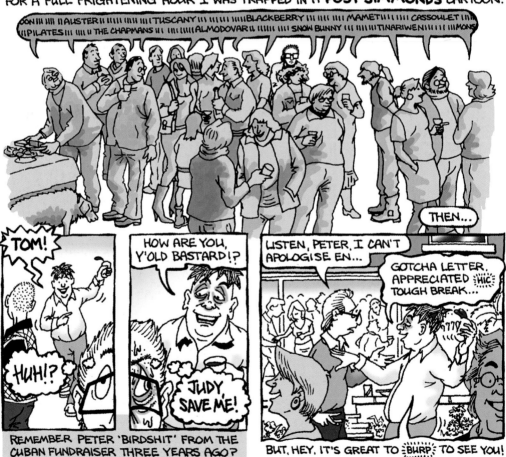

TOM!

HUH!?

HOW ARE YOU, Y'OLD BASTARD!?

JUDY SAVE ME!

REMEMBER PETER 'BIRDSHIT' FROM THE CUBAN FUNDRAISER THREE YEARS AGO?

THEN...

LISTEN, PETER, I CAN'T APOLOGISE EN...

GOTCHA LETTER. APPRECIATED :HIC: TOUGH BREAK...

BUT, HEY, IT'S GREAT TO :BURP: TO SEE YOU!

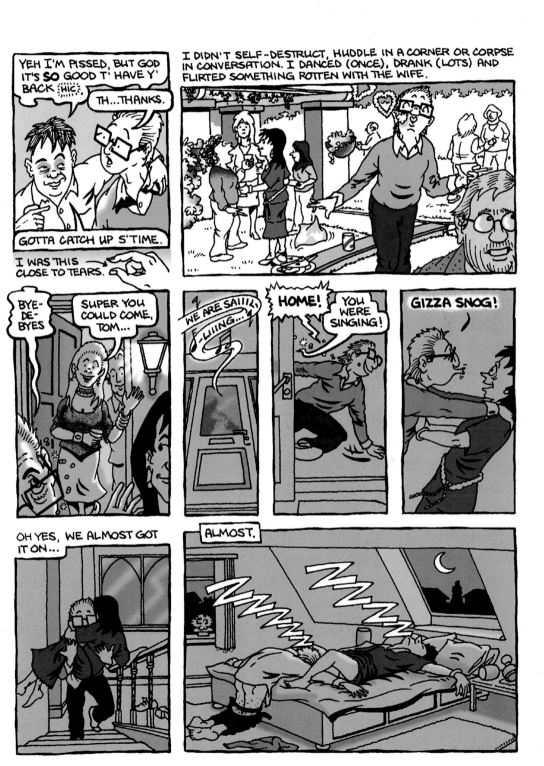

ONE DAY I SURPRISED MYSELF BY GOING FOR A RIDE, NOT TO SHOP OR KEEP AN APPOINTMENT, BUT FOR PLEASURE.

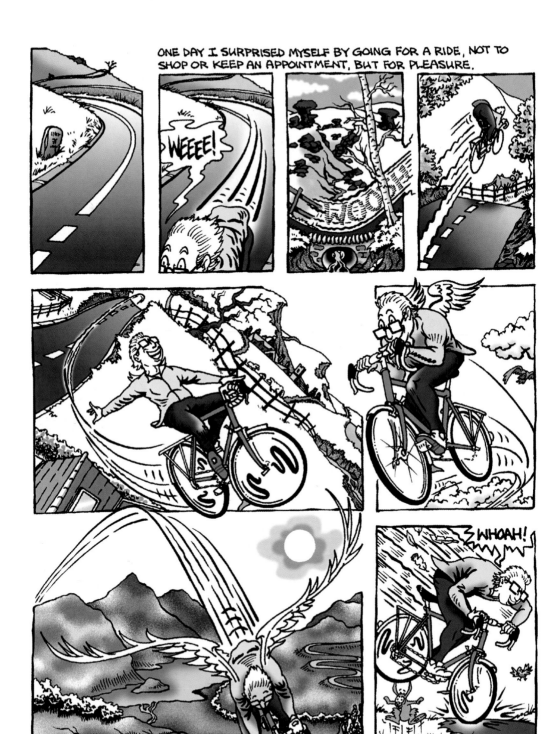

WEEEE!

WHOAH!

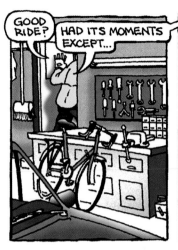

GOOD RIDE?

HAD ITS MOMENTS EXCEPT...

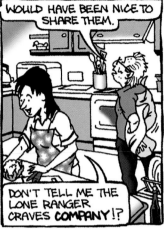

WOULD HAVE BEEN NICE TO SHARE THEM.

DON'T TELL ME THE LONE RANGER CRAVES **COMPANY**!?

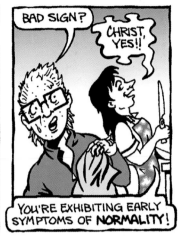

BAD SIGN?

CHRIST, YES!!

YOU'RE EXHIBITING EARLY SYMPTOMS OF **NORMALITY**!

A CHANGE OF PHYSICAL JERKS WAS NEEDED. ON THE BASIS IT WAS HUMAN POWERED, AFFORDED TRAVEL AND REQUIRED ME TO BE SOCIABLE WITH ONLY ONE OTHER PERSON...

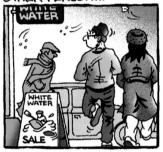

I TOOK UP CANOEING.

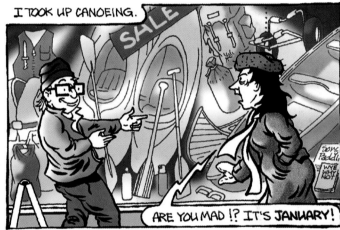

ARE YOU MAD!? IT'S JANUARY!

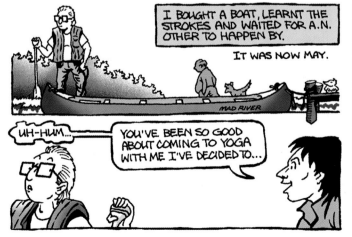

I BOUGHT A BOAT, LEARNT THE STROKES AND WAITED FOR A.N. OTHER TO HAPPEN BY.

IT WAS NOW MAY.

UH-HUM...

YOU'VE BEEN SO GOOD ABOUT COMING TO YOGA WITH ME I'VE DECIDED TO...

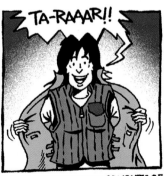

TA-RAAAR!!

DID I MENTION THE ADVANTAGE OF CANOEING OVER CYCLING WITH ANOTHER PERSON IS THAT YOU'RE IN THE SAME BOAT AND CAN'T **COMPETE**?

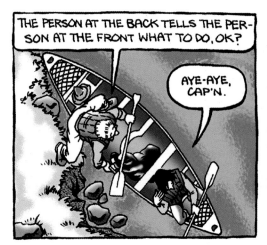

THE PERSON AT THE BACK TELLS THE PERSON AT THE FRONT WHAT TO DO, OK?

AYE-AYE, CAP'N.

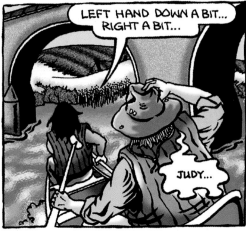

LEFT HAND DOWN A BIT... RIGHT A BIT...

JUDY...

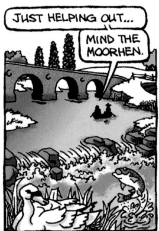

JUST HELPING OUT...

MIND THE MOORHEN.

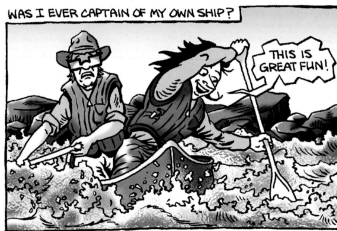

WAS I EVER CAPTAIN OF MY OWN SHIP?

THIS IS GREAT FUN!

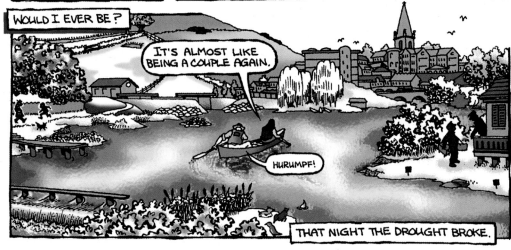

WOULD I EVER BE?

IT'S ALMOST LIKE BEING A COUPLE AGAIN.

HURUMPF!

THAT NIGHT THE DROUGHT BROKE.

228

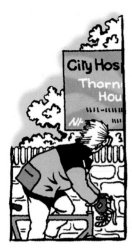

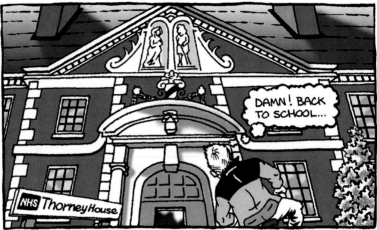

DAMN! BACK TO SCHOOL...

NHS ThorneyHouse

TWO YEARS TO THE MONTH AFTER I SAW DR. MATTERHORN I GOT TO SEE AN NHS PSYCHODYNAMIC PSYCHOTHERAPIST (YOU MIGHT WELL ASK!), A DR. CALLAS.

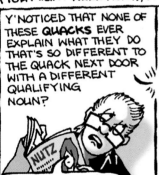

Y'NOTICED THAT NONE OF THESE **QUACKS** EVER EXPLAIN WHAT THEY DO THAT'S SO DIFFERENT TO THE QUACK NEXT DOOR WITH A DIFFERENT QUALIFYING NOUN?

NUTZ

OH, **YOU'RE** HERE.

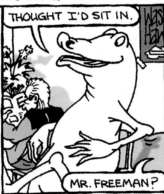

THOUGHT I'D SIT IN.

MR. FREEMAN?

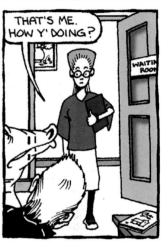

THAT'S ME. HOW Y'DOING?

WAITIN ROOM

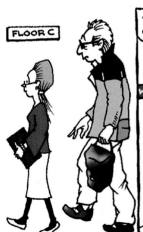

FLOOR C

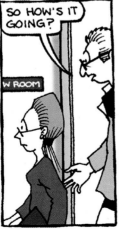

SO HOW'S IT GOING?

W ROOM

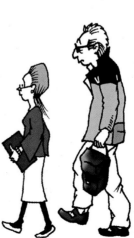

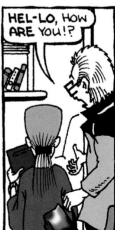

HEL-LO, HOW ARE YOU!?

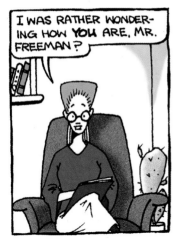

I WAS RATHER WONDERING HOW **YOU** ARE, MR. FREEMAN?

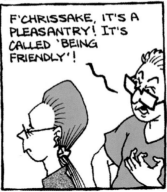

THIS ICY PERFORMANCE WAS REPEATED AT EACH OF MY VISITS UNTIL...

F'CHRISSAKE, IT'S A PLEASANTRY! IT'S CALLED 'BEING FRIENDLY'!

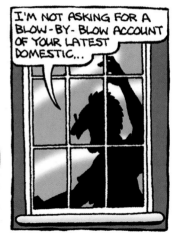

I'M NOT ASKING FOR A BLOW-BY-BLOW ACCOUNT OF YOUR LATEST DOMESTIC...

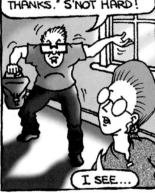

LIE IF YOU HAVE TO. WE ALL DO. "I'M FINE, THANKS." S'NOT HARD!

I SEE...

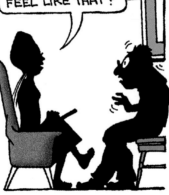

WERE YOU NEGLECTED AS A CHILD OR DOES IT JUST FEEL LIKE THAT?

CALLAS WAS EVIDENTLY A GRADUATE OF THE NURSE RATCHED SCHOOL OF INTER-PERSONAL SKILLS.

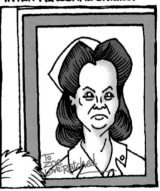

DR. CALLAS WAS A SCRIBBLER. I ONLY HAD TO LOOK AWAY AND IT WAS IN HER NOTES, LOGGED AND TIMED.

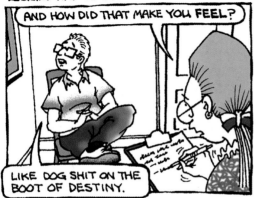

AND HOW DID THAT MAKE YOU **FEEL**?

LIKE DOG SHIT ON THE BOOT OF DESTINY.

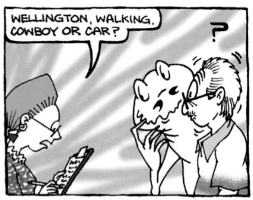

WELLINGTON, WALKING, COWBOY OR CAR?

?

SHE SCRUTINIZED MY RESPONSES LIKE EACH WAS A CRIME SCENE, BUT THEN I WAS BEING ASSESSED...

...BY A SHRINK WHO DRIPPED CONDESCENSION LIKE A TRANSPORT CAFÉ CEILING.

ER... THAT'S CONDENSATION.

SHHH... I'M THINKING.

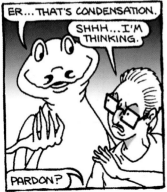

PARDON?

YOU ASKED WHAT ALBUMS I BOUGHT.

YES.

DARED I ADMIT, A COUPLE BY KATE BUSH? I WAS DOING THE OH-SO ENGLISH—**KINKS,** BEATLES, BLUR...

A COUPLE BY ANTHRAX, WHY?

....

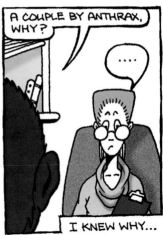

I KNEW WHY...

WE WERE PLAYING **MIND-GAMES,** AND HAD BEEN SINCE MY TOLERANCE FOR BEING QUESTIONED LIKE HER FAVOURITE SON EVAPORATED TEN MINUTES INTO SESSION TWO.

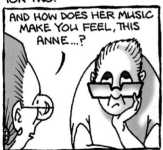

AND HOW DOES HER MUSIC MAKE YOU FEEL, THIS ANNE...?

I WOULD HAVE WALKED OUT, HAD A VISION OF **JOB CENTRE GARETH** NOT COME CHARGING IN.

GREAT NEWS, TOM...

ALL I NEEDED WAS HER COMPUTER TELLING HIS COMPUTER I HAD 'REJECTED TREATMENT' AND...

LIDL HAVE A VACANCY!!

IT TOOK FIVE INTERROGATIONS SPREAD OVER AS MANY MONTHS FOR A COVEN OF PSYCHOLOGISTS, PSYCHIATRISTS, SUNDRY THERAPISTS AND A PASSING CARETAKER TO CONCLUDE....

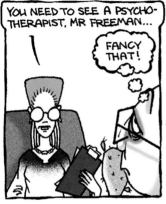

YOU NEED TO SEE A PSYCHO-THERAPIST, MR FREEMAN...

FANCY THAT!

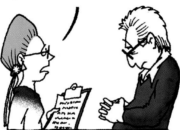

AND THERE'S EVERY CHANCE WE CAN FIND YOU AN APPOINTMENT BEFORE NEXT YEAR, UNLESS YOU HAVE A GENDER PREFERENCE...

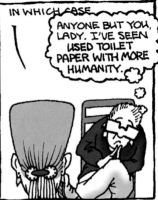

IN WHICH CASE...

ANYONE BUT YOU, LADY. I'VE SEEN USED TOILET PAPER WITH MORE HUMANITY.

231

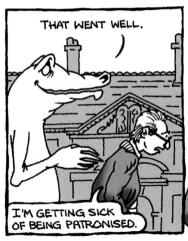

THAT WENT WELL.

I'M GETTING SICK OF BEING PATRONISED.

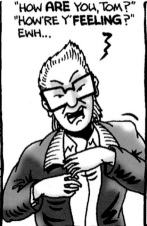

"HOW **ARE** YOU, TOM?" "HOW'RE Y'**FEELING**?" EWH...

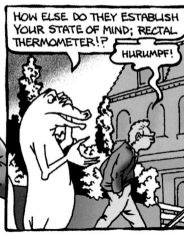

HOW ELSE DO THEY ESTABLISH YOUR STATE OF MIND; RECTAL THERMOMETER!?

HURUMPF!

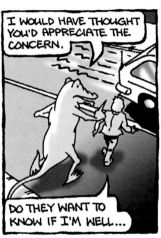

I WOULD HAVE THOUGHT YOU'D APPRECIATE THE CONCERN.

DO THEY WANT TO KNOW IF I'M WELL...

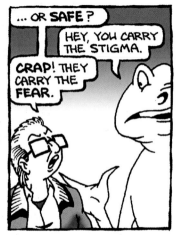

... OR **SAFE**?

HEY, YOU CARRY THE STIGMA.

CRAP! THEY CARRY THE FEAR.

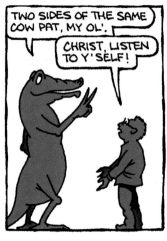

TWO SIDES OF THE SAME COW PAT, MY OL'.

CHRIST, LISTEN TO Y'SELF!

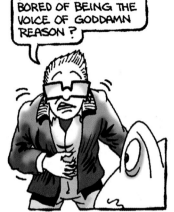

DON'T YOU EVER GET BORED OF BEING THE VOICE OF GODDAMN REASON?

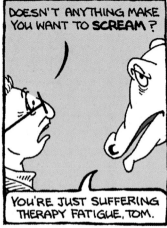

DOESN'T ANYTHING MAKE YOU WANT TO **SCREAM**?

YOU'RE JUST SUFFERING THERAPY FATIGUE, TOM.

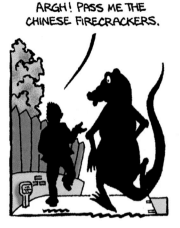

ARGH! PASS ME THE CHINESE FIRECRACKERS.

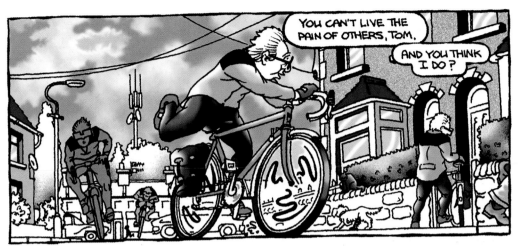

YOU CAN'T LIVE THE PAIN OF OTHERS, TOM.

AND YOU THINK I DO?

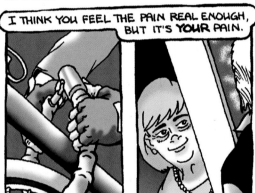

I THINK YOU FEEL THE PAIN REAL ENOUGH, BUT IT'S **YOUR** PAIN.

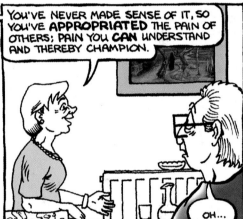

YOU'VE NEVER MADE SENSE OF IT, SO YOU'VE **APPROPRIATED** THE PAIN OF OTHERS; PAIN YOU **CAN** UNDERSTAND AND THEREBY CHAMPION.

OH...

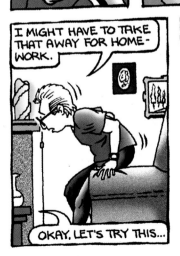

I MIGHT HAVE TO TAKE THAT AWAY FOR HOMEWORK.

OKAY, LET'S TRY THIS...

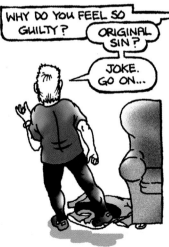

WHY DO YOU FEEL SO GUILTY?

ORIGINAL SIN?

JOKE. GO ON...

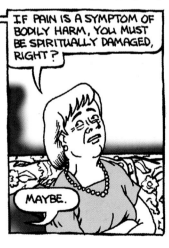

IF PAIN IS A SYMPTOM OF BODILY HARM, YOU MUST BE SPIRITUALLY DAMAGED, RIGHT?

MAYBE.

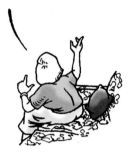

SOME TERRIBLE WRONG HAS BEEN COMMITTED, YOU THINK BY YOU. YOU DON'T KNOW WHAT, WHEN OR HOW, BUT YOU FEEL GUILTY AS SIN.

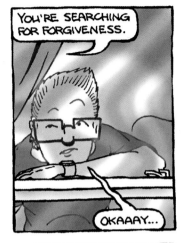

YOU'RE SEARCHING FOR FORGIVENESS.

OKAAAY...

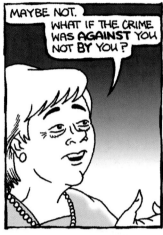

MAYBE NOT. WHAT IF THE CRIME WAS **AGAINST** YOU NOT **BY** YOU?

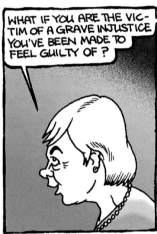

WHAT IF YOU ARE THE VIC-TIM OF A GRAVE INJUSTICE YOU'VE BEEN MADE TO FEEL GUILTY OF?

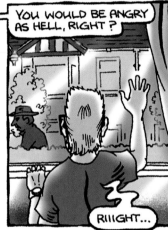

YOU WOULD BE ANGRY AS HELL, RIGHT?

RIIIGHT...

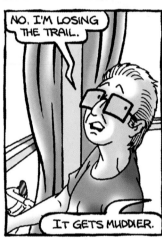

NO, I'M LOSING THE TRAIL.

IT GETS MUDDIER.

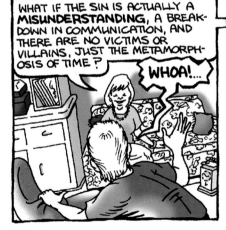

WHAT IF THE SIN IS ACTUALLY A **MISUNDERSTANDING**, A BREAK-DOWN IN COMMUNICATION, AND THERE ARE NO VICTIMS OR VILLAINS, JUST THE METAMORPH-OSIS OF TIME?

WHOA!....

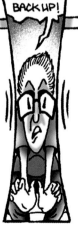

BACK UP!

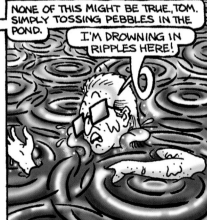

NONE OF THIS MIGHT BE TRUE, TOM. SIMPLY TOSSING PEBBLES IN THE POND.

I'M DROWNING IN RIPPLES HERE!

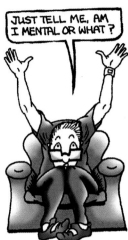

JUST TELL ME, AM I MENTAL OR WHAT?

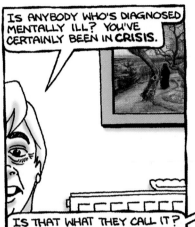

IS ANYBODY WHO'S DIAGNOSED MENTALLY ILL? YOU'VE CERTAINLY BEEN IN **CRISIS**.

IS THAT WHAT THEY CALL IT?

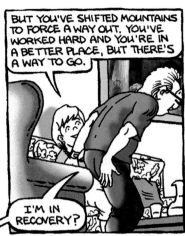

BUT YOU'VE SHIFTED MOUNTAINS TO FORCE A WAY OUT. YOU'VE WORKED HARD AND YOU'RE IN A BETTER PLACE, BUT THERE'S A WAY TO GO.

I'M IN RECOVERY?

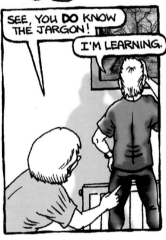

SEE, YOU **DO** KNOW THE JARGON!

I'M LEARNING.

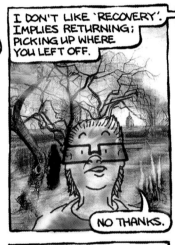

I DON'T LIKE 'RECOVERY'. IMPLIES RETURNING; PICKING UP WHERE YOU LEFT OFF.

NO THANKS.

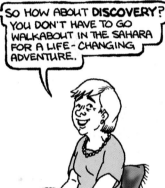

SO HOW ABOUT **DISCOVERY**? YOU DON'T HAVE TO GO WALKABOUT IN THE SAHARA FOR A LIFE-CHANGING ADVENTURE.

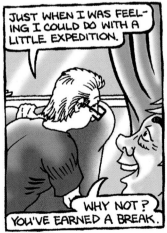

JUST WHEN I WAS FEELING I COULD DO WITH A LITTLE EXPEDITION.

WHY NOT? YOU'VE EARNED A BREAK.

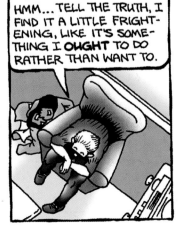

HMM... TELL THE TRUTH, I FIND IT A LITTLE FRIGHTENING, LIKE IT'S SOMETHING I **OUGHT** TO DO RATHER THAN WANT TO.

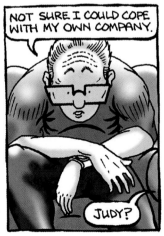

NOT SURE I COULD COPE WITH MY OWN COMPANY.

JUDY?

235

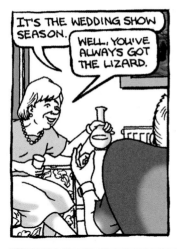

IT'S THE WEDDING SHOW SEASON.

WELL, YOU'VE ALWAYS GOT THE LIZARD.

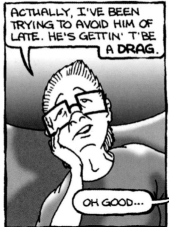

ACTUALLY, I'VE BEEN TRYING TO AVOID HIM OF LATE. HE'S GETTIN' T'BE A DRAG.

OH GOOD...

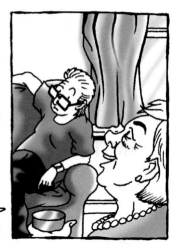

IT WAS TO BE MY LAST - BUT-ONE SESSION WITH DR. SUSAN HUGG.

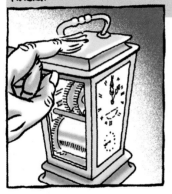

THE MONEY RAN OUT. THE FREEMAN HOUSEHOLD WAS NOW OFFICIALLY BANKRUPT.

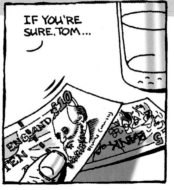

IF YOU'RE SURE, TOM...

HUGG OFFERED TO CONTINUE WITH NO FEE, BUT I COULDN'T DO THAT.
I KNEW HER WORTH.

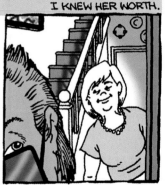

BESIDES, I WAS ON THE FINAL RUN INTO SEE AN N.H.S. SHRINK, AND WHO WAS TO SAY THEY WOULDN'T BE JUST AS BRILLIANT AS SUSAN HUGG?

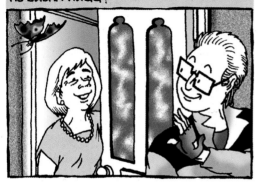

SO...'YOU GOT SOMETHING YOU WANT TO SAY?

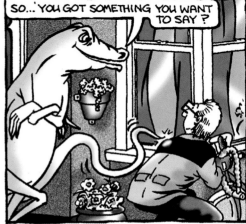

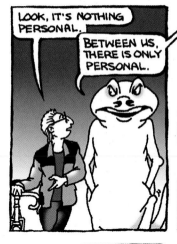

LOOK, IT'S NOTHING PERSONAL.

BETWEEN US, THERE IS ONLY PERSONAL.

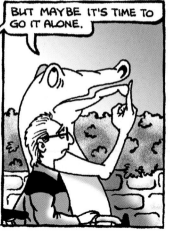

BUT MAYBE IT'S TIME TO GO IT ALONE.

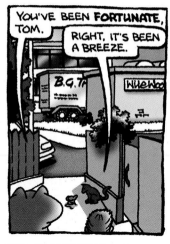

YOU'VE BEEN **FORTUNATE**, TOM.

RIGHT, IT'S BEEN A BREEZE.

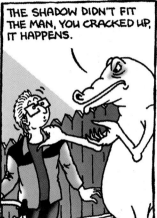

THE SHADOW DIDN'T FIT THE MAN, YOU CRACKED UP, IT HAPPENS.

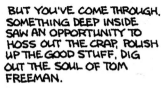
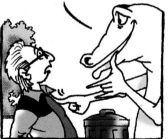

BUT YOU'VE COME THROUGH. SOMETHING DEEP INSIDE SAW AN OPPORTUNITY TO HOSS OUT THE CRAP, POLISH UP THE GOOD STUFF, DIG OUT THE SOUL OF TOM FREEMAN.

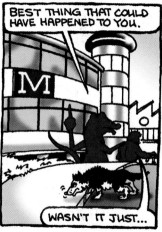

BEST THING THAT COULD HAVE HAPPENED TO YOU.

WASN'T IT JUST...

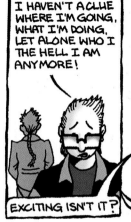

I HAVEN'T A CLUE WHERE I'M GOING, WHAT I'M DOING, LET ALONE WHO I THE HELL I AM ANYMORE!

EXCITING ISN'T IT?

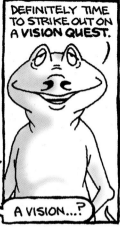

DEFINITELY TIME TO STRIKE OUT ON A **VISION QUEST**.

A VISION...?

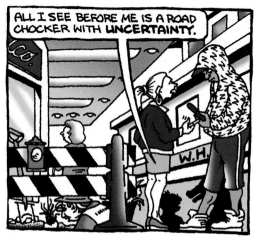

ALL I SEE BEFORE ME IS A ROAD CHOCKER WITH **UNCERTAINTY**.

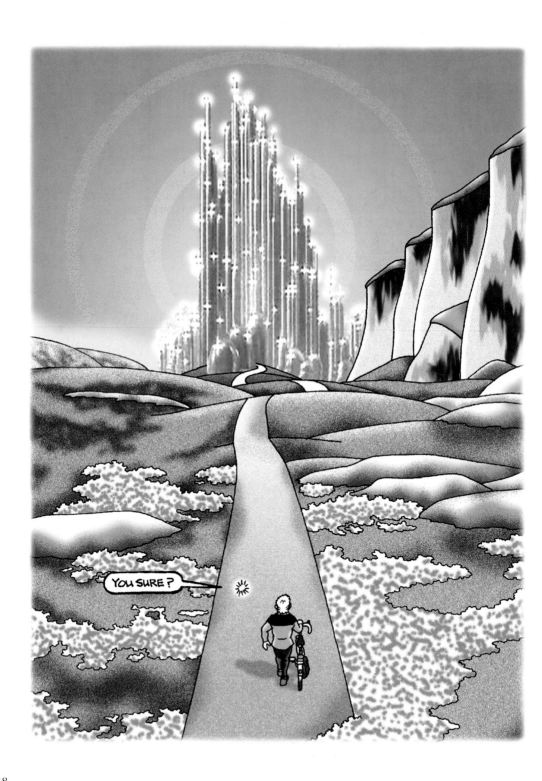

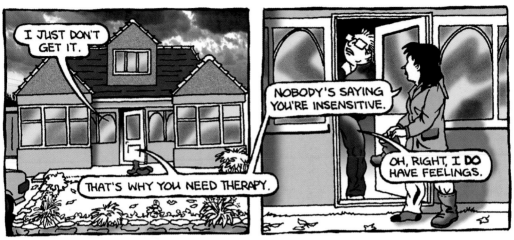

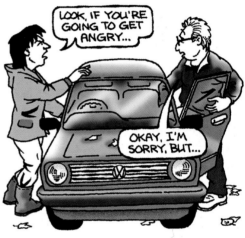

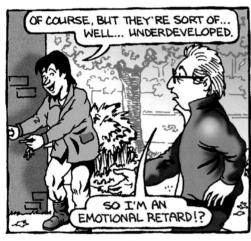

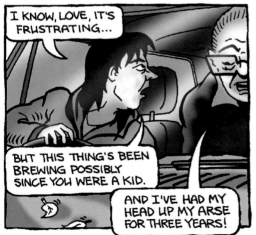

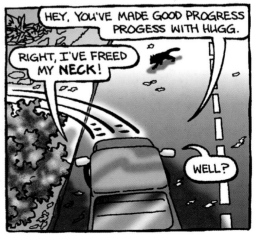

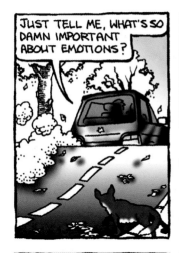

JUST TELL ME, WHAT'S SO DAMN IMPORTANT ABOUT EMOTIONS?

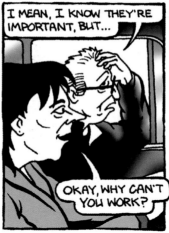

I MEAN, I KNOW THEY'RE IMPORTANT, BUT...

OKAY, WHY CAN'T YOU WORK?

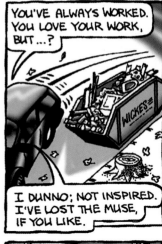

YOU'VE ALWAYS WORKED. YOU LOVE YOUR WORK, BUT...?

I DUNNO; NOT INSPIRED. I'VE LOST THE MUSE, IF YOU LIKE.

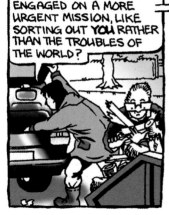

OR ARE YOU OTHERWISE ENGAGED ON A MORE URGENT MISSION, LIKE SORTING OUT **YOU** RATHER THAN THE TROUBLES OF THE WORLD?

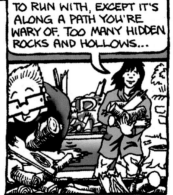

I THINK HUGG'S SET A BALL ROLLING YOU WANT TO RUN WITH, EXCEPT IT'S ALONG A PATH YOU'RE WARY OF. TOO MANY HIDDEN ROCKS AND HOLLOWS...

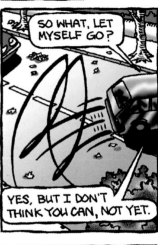

SO WHAT, LET MYSELF GO?

YES, BUT I DON'T THINK YOU CAN, NOT YET.

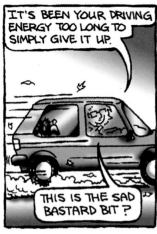

IT'S BEEN YOUR DRIVING ENERGY TOO LONG TO SIMPLY GIVE IT UP.

THIS IS THE SAD BASTARD BIT?

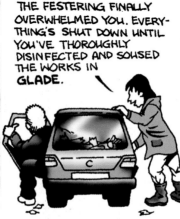

THE FESTERING FINALLY OVERWHELMED YOU. EVERYTHING'S SHUT DOWN UNTIL YOU'VE THOROUGHLY DISINFECTED AND SOUSED THE WORKS IN **GLADE.**

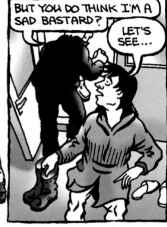

BUT YOU DO THINK I'M A SAD BASTARD?

LET'S SEE...

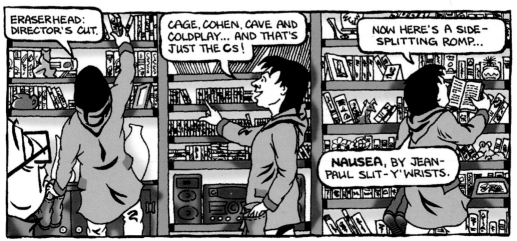

ERASERHEAD: DIRECTOR'S CUT.

CAGE, COHEN, CAVE AND COLDPLAY... AND THAT'S JUST THE Cs!

NOW HERE'S A SIDE-SPLITTING ROMP...

NAUSEA, BY JEAN-PAUL SLIT-Y'WRISTS.

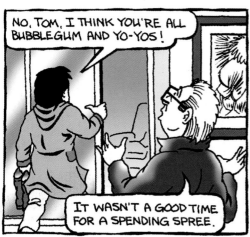

NO, TOM, I THINK YOU'RE ALL BUBBLEGUM AND YO-YOS!

IT WASN'T A GOOD TIME FOR A SPENDING SPREE.

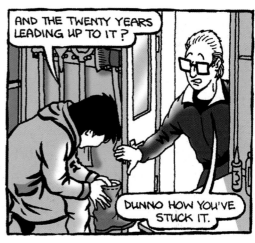

AND THE TWENTY YEARS LEADING UP TO IT?

DUNNO HOW YOU'VE STUCK IT.

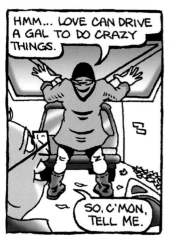

HMM... LOVE CAN DRIVE A GAL TO DO CRAZY THINGS.

SO, C'MON, TELL ME.

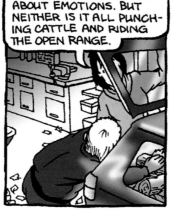

I DON'T THINK IT IS ALL ABOUT EMOTIONS. BUT NEITHER IS IT ALL PUNCH-ING CATTLE AND RIDING THE OPEN RANGE.

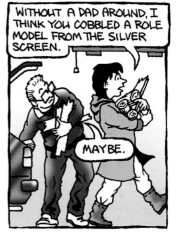

WITHOUT A DAD AROUND, I THINK YOU COBBLED A ROLE MODEL FROM THE SILVER SCREEN.

MAYBE.

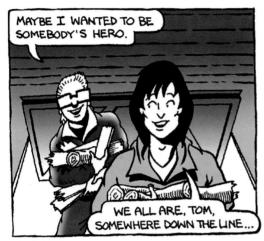

MAYBE I WANTED TO BE SOMEBODY'S HERO.

WE ALL ARE, TOM, SOMEWHERE DOWN THE LINE...

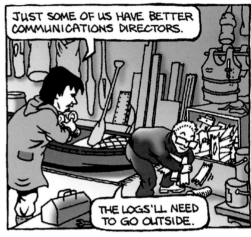

JUST SOME OF US HAVE BETTER COMMUNICATIONS DIRECTORS.

THE LOGS'LL NEED TO GO OUTSIDE.

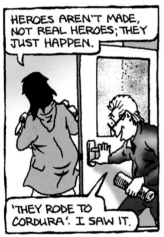

HEROES AREN'T MADE, NOT REAL HEROES; THEY JUST HAPPEN.

'THEY RODE TO CORDURA'. I SAW IT.

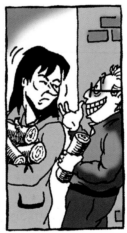

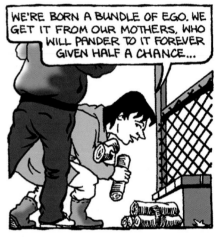

WE'RE BORN A BUNDLE OF EGO. WE GET IT FROM OUR MOTHERS, WHO WILL PANDER TO IT FOREVER GIVEN HALF A CHANCE...

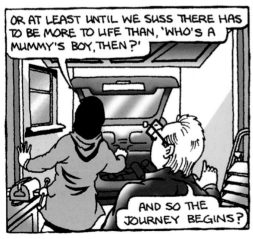

OR AT LEAST UNTIL WE SUSS THERE HAS TO BE MORE TO LIFE THAN, 'WHO'S A MUMMY'S BOY, THEN?'

AND SO THE JOURNEY BEGINS?

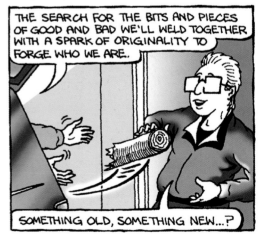

THE SEARCH FOR THE BITS AND PIECES OF GOOD AND BAD WE'LL WELD TOGETHER WITH A SPARK OF ORIGINALITY TO FORGE WHO WE ARE.

SOMETHING OLD, SOMETHING NEW...?

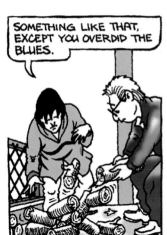

SOMETHING LIKE THAT, EXCEPT YOU OVERDID THE BLUES.

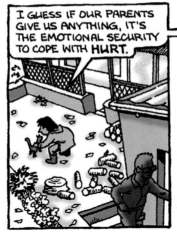

I GUESS IF OUR PARENTS GIVE US ANYTHING, IT'S THE EMOTIONAL SECURITY TO COPE WITH **HURT.**

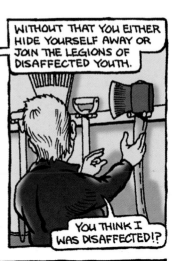

WITHOUT THAT YOU EITHER HIDE YOURSELF AWAY OR JOIN THE LEGIONS OF DISAFFECTED YOUTH.

YOU THINK I WAS DISAFFECTED!?

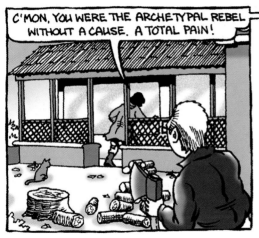

C'MON, YOU WERE THE ARCHETYPAL REBEL WITHOUT A CAUSE. A TOTAL PAIN!

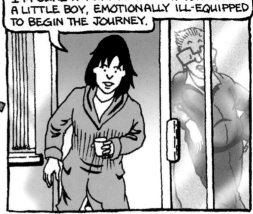

YOU SET OUT TO **REPULSE** PEOPLE; STRAIGHTS. NOT JUST THE SNOTS YOU MET AT SCHOOL, BUT ANYBODY VAGUELY RESPECTABLE.

IT'S WHAT OUR GENERATION DID!

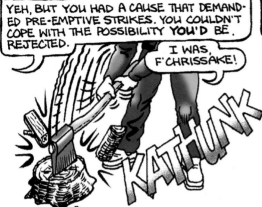

YEH, BUT YOU HAD A CAUSE THAT DEMANDED PRE-EMPTIVE STRIKES. YOU COULDN'T COPE WITH THE POSSIBILITY **YOU'D** BE REJECTED.

I WAS, F'CHRISSAKE!

KATHUNK

I'M SURE IT FELT LIKE THAT. YOU WERE A LITTLE BOY, EMOTIONALLY ILL-EQUIPPED TO BEGIN THE JOURNEY.

243

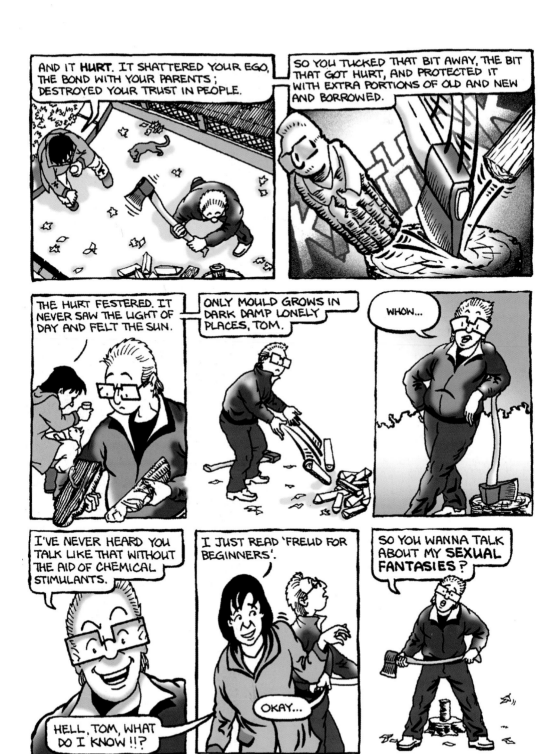

AND IT **HURT**. IT SHATTERED YOUR EGO, THE BOND WITH YOUR PARENTS; DESTROYED YOUR TRUST IN PEOPLE.

SO YOU TUCKED THAT BIT AWAY, THE BIT THAT GOT HURT, AND PROTECTED IT WITH EXTRA PORTIONS OF OLD AND NEW AND BORROWED.

THE HURT FESTERED. IT NEVER SAW THE LIGHT OF DAY AND FELT THE SUN.

ONLY MOULD GROWS IN DARK DAMP LONELY PLACES, TOM.

WHOW...

I'VE NEVER HEARD YOU TALK LIKE THAT WITHOUT THE AID OF CHEMICAL STIMULANTS.

HELL, TOM, WHAT DO I KNOW !!?

I JUST READ 'FREUD FOR BEGINNERS'.

OKAY...

SO YOU WANNA TALK ABOUT MY **SEXUAL FANTASIES**?

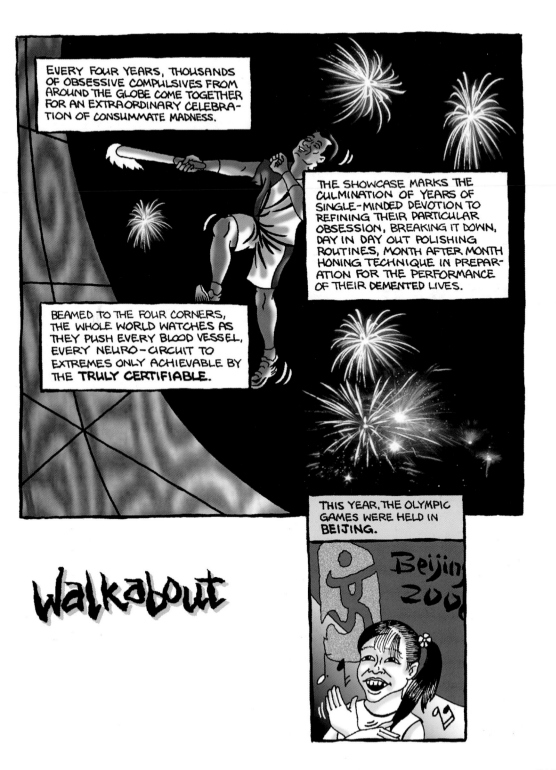

EVERY FOUR YEARS, THOUSANDS OF OBSESSIVE COMPULSIVES FROM AROUND THE GLOBE COME TOGETHER FOR AN EXTRAORDINARY CELEBRATION OF CONSUMMATE MADNESS.

THE SHOWCASE MARKS THE CULMINATION OF YEARS OF SINGLE-MINDED DEVOTION TO REFINING THEIR PARTICULAR OBSESSION, BREAKING IT DOWN, DAY IN DAY OUT POLISHING ROUTINES, MONTH AFTER MONTH HONING TECHNIQUE IN PREPARATION FOR THE PERFORMANCE OF THEIR DEMENTED LIVES.

BEAMED TO THE FOUR CORNERS, THE WHOLE WORLD WATCHES AS THEY PUSH EVERY BLOOD VESSEL, EVERY NEURO-CIRCUIT TO EXTREMES ONLY ACHIEVABLE BY THE **TRULY CERTIFIABLE.**

Walkabout

THIS YEAR, THE OLYMPIC GAMES WERE HELD IN **BEIJING.**

Beijing 200

I FILLED THE FRIDGE, STOCKED UP ON SIX-PACKS AND BOLTED MYSELF TO THE TUBE.

IT WAS AN OPPORTUNITY NOT TO BE MISSED, FOR THE BBC AS MUCH THE PRC. *

THE VOICE OF STATE BROADCASTING WAS HUW EDWARDS, A NEWSCASTER NOT A SPORTSCASTER.

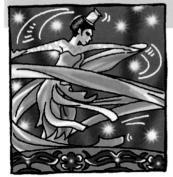

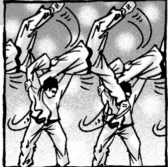

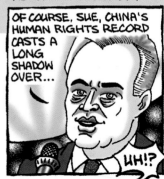

OF COURSE, SUE, CHINA'S HUMAN RIGHTS RECORD CASTS A LONG SHADOW OVER...

UH!?

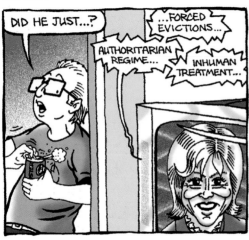

DID HE JUST...?

...FORCED EVICTIONS...

AUTHORITARIAN REGIME...

INHUMAN TREATMENT...

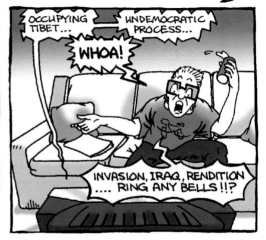

OCCUPYING TIBET...

UNDEMOCRATIC PROCESS...

WHOA!

INVASION, IRAQ, RENDITION.... RING ANY BELLS !!?

IT WAS TOO GOOD A JOKE NOT TO **SHARE**.

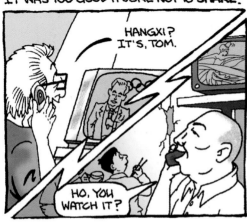

HANGXI? IT'S, TOM.

HO, YOU WATCH IT?

I TOLD HIM TEAM G.B.'S LINE, COMPLETE WITH WELSH ACCENT.

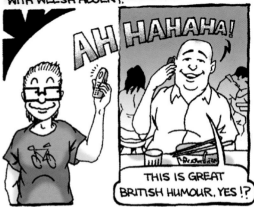

AH HAHAHA!

THIS IS GREAT BRITISH HUMOUR, YES !?

* PEOPLE'S REPUBLIC OF CHINA

IT GOT **FUNNIER** AS THE SHOW UNFOLDED. SUDDENLY IT WAS...

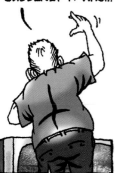

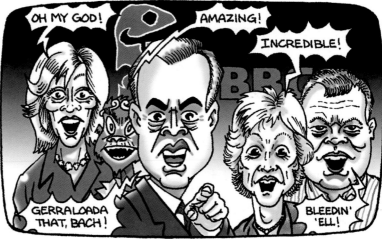

OH MY GOD!

AMAZING!

INCREDIBLE!

GERRALOADA THAT, BACH!

BLEEDIN' 'ELL!

THEN...

OF COURSE, SUE, LONDON 2012 DOESN'T HAVE TO BEAT THAT.

SOMETHING LESS SHOWY.

THE GREEN GAMES...

BACK TO BASICS...

BEEFEATERS, MORRIS MEN AND PEARLY QUEENS!

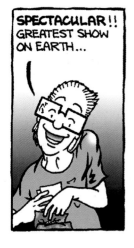

THEY'RE SHITTING THEMSELVES!

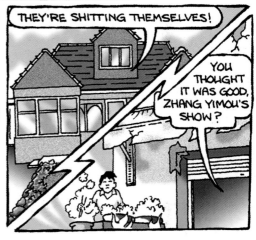

YOU THOUGHT IT WAS GOOD, ZHANG YIMOU'S SHOW?

SPECTACULAR!! GREATEST SHOW ON EARTH...

WE DID NOT LIKE IT. TOO MUCH HE KOWTOWED TO WESTERN STEREO- TYPE OF CHINA.

THOSE DAMN DYNASTIC TRADIT- IONS, EH, BUT NO MAO?

SEE HOW MANY PERFORMERS.

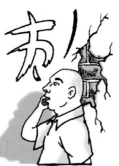

I SAY NOTHING EXCEPT...

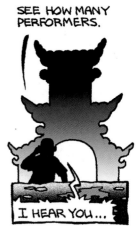

I HEAR YOU...

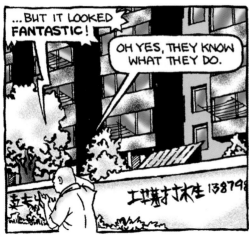

...BUT IT LOOKED **FANTASTIC!**

OH YES, THEY KNOW WHAT THEY DO.

工峰打木生 13879

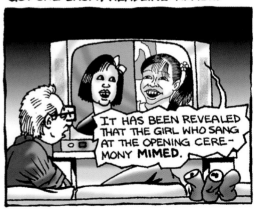

A COUPLE OF DAYS LATER, THE WEST GOT ONE BACK. HEADLINE NEWS...

IT HAS BEEN REVEALED THAT THE GIRL WHO SANG AT THE OPENING CERE-MONY **MIMED.**

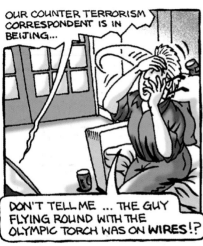

OUR COUNTER TERRORISM CORRESPONDENT IS IN BEIJING...

DON'T TELL ME ... THE GUY FLYING ROUND WITH THE OLYMPIC TORCH WAS ON **WIRES!?**

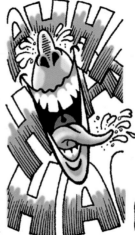

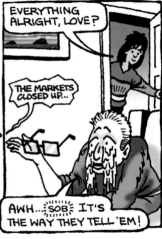

EVERYTHING ALRIGHT, LOVE?

THE MARKETS CLOSED UP...

AWH... SOB IT'S THE WAY THEY TELL 'EM!

THE FUN AND GAMES JUST GOT **BETTER.** WITHIN A COUPLE OF MONTHS EVERYBODY WAS TALKING SUB-PRIMES, CREDIT CRUNCH AND GLOBAL MARKET MELTDOWN.

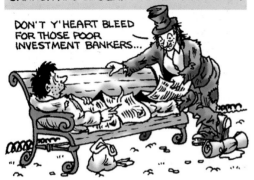

DON'T Y'HEART BLEED FOR THOSE POOR INVESTMENT BANKERS...

BOY RACERS IN THE BOWELS OF THE MACHINE HAD DRIVEN THE ENGINE OF CAPITALISM TO A STANDSTILL.

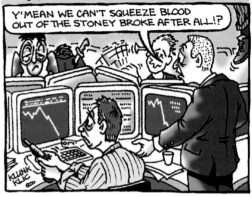

Y'MEAN WE CAN'T SQUEEZE BLOOD OUT OF THE STONEY BROKE AFTER ALL!?

KLUNK KLIC

BANKS WENT BELLY UP, ECONOMIES SKIDDED TO A HALT AND GOVERNMENTS RUSHED TO THE RESCUE OF OLD SCHOOL CHUMS, FLOODING THE ENGINE WITH TAXPAYERS' BILLIONS (LIKE MORE OIL HAS EVER FREED UP A SEIZED ENGINE!).

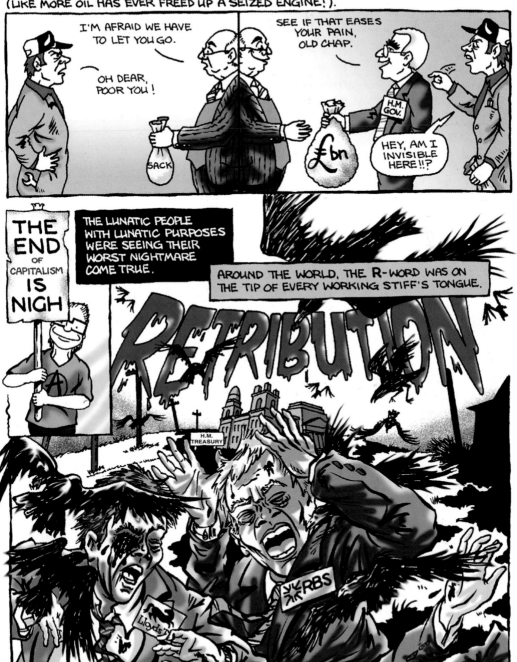

BUT, HALLELUJAH, A NEW **MESSIAH** RODE IN FROM THE WEST PREACHING A SERMON OF HOPE. AS FAR AFIELD AS KISUMU, KENYA, THERE WAS DANCING IN THE STREETS.

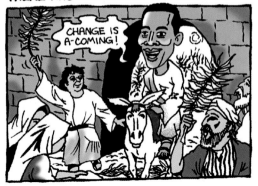

A RICH BLACK MAN REPLACED A RICH WHITE MAN (PART APE) AT THE HELM OF THE AMERICAN SUPERTANKER STEAMING FOR THE ROCKS.

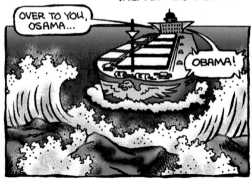

AND GUESS WHO THE **USS UNCLE SAM** S.O.S.ED FOR HELP?

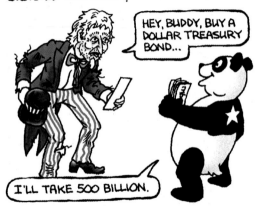

THE WORLD WAS GOING **BONKERS.** SUDDENLY THE FUNNIEST SHOW ON AIR WAS THE **NEWS.**

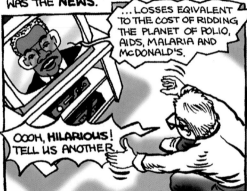

IN THE SAME MONTH UNEMPLOYMENT HIT A 70 YEAR HIGH...

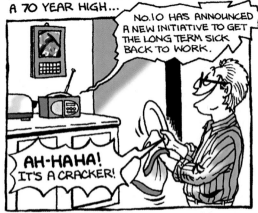

IN THE SAME WEEK BANKER BONUSES IN THE **BILLIONS** WERE CONFIRMED, THE JOBCENTRE QUESTIONED MY (NOW) 80 QUID A WEEK BENEFIT.

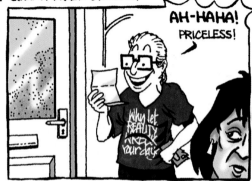

250

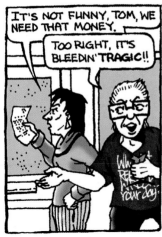

IT'S NOT FUNNY, TOM, WE NEED THAT MONEY.

TOO RIGHT, IT'S BLEEDIN' **TRAGIC**!!

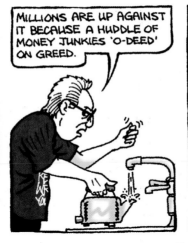

MILLIONS ARE UP AGAINST IT BECAUSE A HUDDLE OF MONEY JUNKIES 'O-DEED' ON GREED.

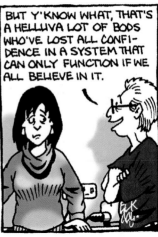

BUT Y'KNOW WHAT, THAT'S A HELLUVA LOT OF BODS WHO'VE LOST ALL CONFIDENCE IN A SYSTEM THAT CAN ONLY FUNCTION IF WE ALL BELIEVE IN IT.

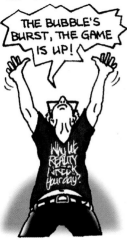

THE BUBBLE'S BURST, THE GAME IS UP!

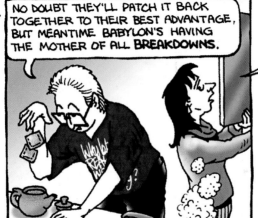

NO DOUBT THEY'LL PATCH IT BACK TOGETHER TO THEIR BEST ADVANTAGE, BUT MEANTIME BABYLON'S HAVING THE MOTHER OF ALL **BREAKDOWNS**.

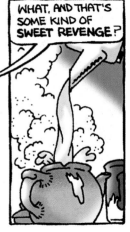

WHAT, AND THAT'S SOME KIND OF **SWEET REVENGE**.?

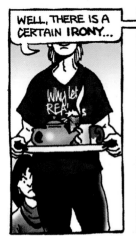

WELL, THERE IS A CERTAIN **IRONY**...

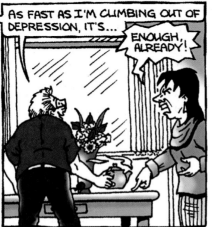

AS FAST AS I'M CLIMBING OUT OF DEPRESSION, IT'S...

ENOUGH, ALREADY!

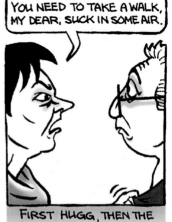

YOU NEED TO TAKE A WALK, MY DEAR, SUCK IN SOME AIR.

FIRST HUGG, THEN THE LIZARD, NOW JUDY...

I STARTED THE WALK IN THE SCOTTISH BORDERS AND PLANNED TO END IT THREE WEEKS AND 338 MILES LATER AT MY DOORSTEP.

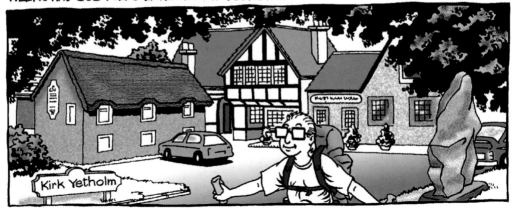

OKAY, IT WAS A LITTLE FURTHER THAN JUDY HAD IN MIND, BUT I NEEDED THE HEAD SPACE.

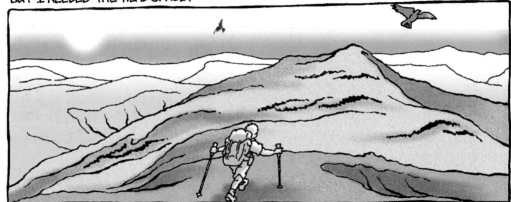

AT BEST, THE PENNINE WAY IS A LONG SLOG DOWN THE BLEAK BACKBONE OF ENGLAND, BUT IF THE SKYLARKS ARE SINGING...

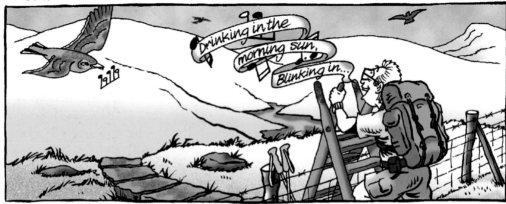

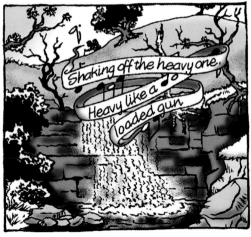

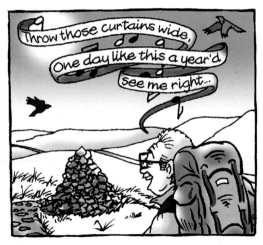

I HAD THREE BEFORE...

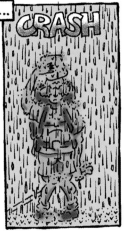

JUST MY LUCK, I HIT THE BRITISH MON-SOON SEASON, THE WORST OF TIMES TO BE ON EXPOSED REACHES.

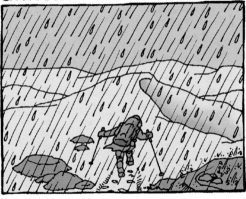

WINDS BLEW AND CRACKED THEIR CHEEKS, RAINS RAN THE GAMUT FROM TORRENTIAL TO BIBLICAL.

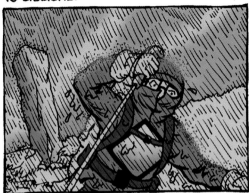

THE MOORS WOBBLED AND OOZED LIKE A PUNCTURED WATER BED. I NEEDED SEA-LEGS!

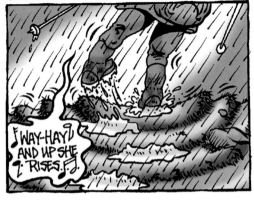

SUDDENLY GLORIOUS PANORAMAS WERE GRIEVOUSLY CROPPED...

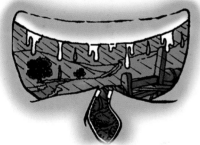

AND ALL I COULD HEAR WAS THE POUNDING OF RAIN ABOVE THE HISSSS OF TINNITUS.

I HAD NEVER FELT SO BOXED IN IN A WILDERNESS.

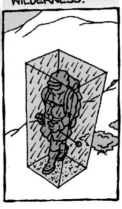

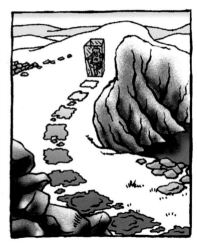

I WAS WITH HUGG FOR A YEAR. WE ROLLED BACK SOME BOULDERS, EVICTED A FEW MONSTERS, BUT THERE WAS MORE TO UNCOVER, PROBABLY MUCH MORE.

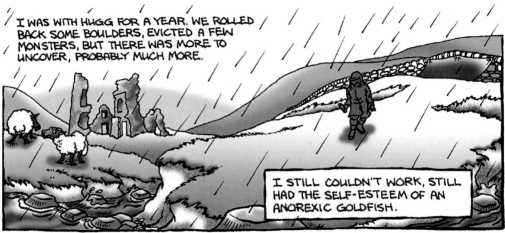

I STILL COULDN'T WORK, STILL HAD THE SELF-ESTEEM OF AN ANOREXIC GOLDFISH.

GLOBS OF ANGER STILL STUCK IN MY CRAW AND, PERVERSELY, I HAD FRESHENED UP THE GUILT.

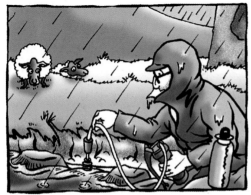

FOUR YEARS HAD BEEN LOST TO A CONDITION IT WAS HARD TO ACCEPT I HADN'T BROUGHT ON MYSELF...

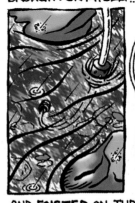

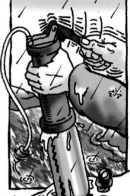

AND **FOISTED** ON JUDY.

254

I'D BLOWN OUR SAVINGS. WE WERE DOWN TO ORANGE-DOT GROCERIES AND CHARITY SHOP LUXURIES.

ON THE OTHER HAND, MY SENSE OF HUMOUR WAS BACK, I WAS MORE LOVED UP THAN EROS ON OYSTERS, AND I HAD SHAKEN THE DAMN LIZARD, FINGERS CROSSED.

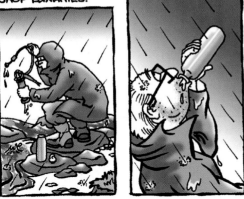

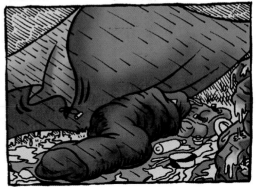

NO THANKS TO THE HEALTH SERVICE, TIME WAS PROVING SOME KIND OF HEALER.

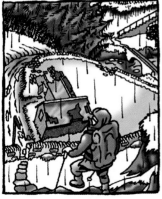

EXCEPT, SOMEWHERE NEAR BOWES, I FELT DISGUST-INGLY ILL.

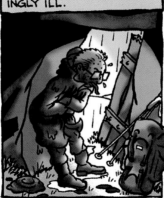

STUFF STARTED POURING OUT OF EVERY ORIFICE.

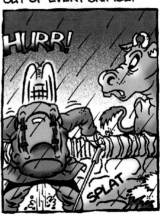

HURR!

SPLAT

I DROPPED MY GUTS REGULAR AS MILE MARKERS.

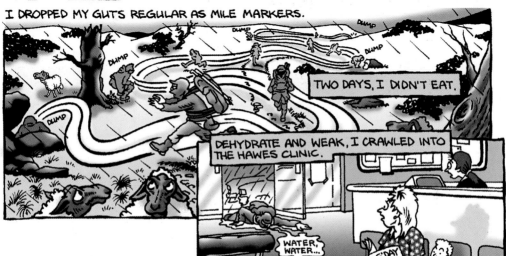

TWO DAYS, I DIDN'T EAT.

DEHYDRATE AND WEAK, I CRAWLED INTO THE HAWES CLINIC.

WATER, WATER...

G'DAY

255

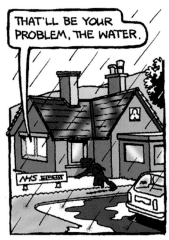

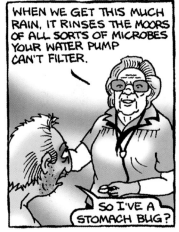

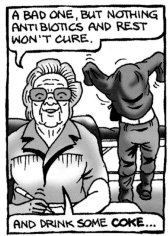

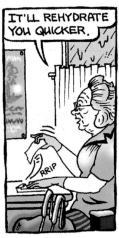

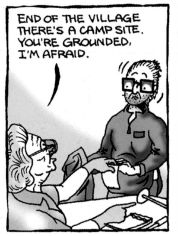

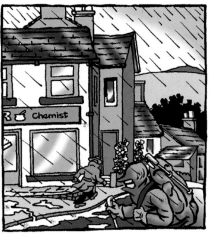

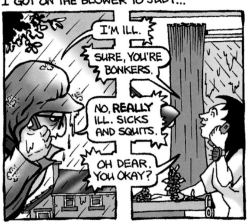

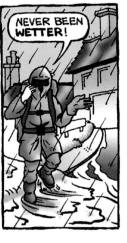

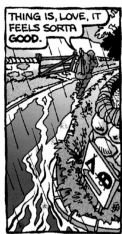

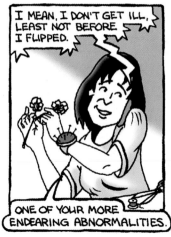

I MEAN, I DON'T GET ILL, LEAST NOT BEFORE I FLIPPED.

ONE OF YOUR MORE ENDEARING ABNORMALITIES.

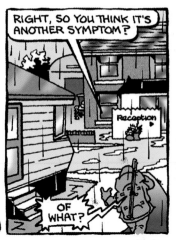

RIGHT, SO YOU THINK IT'S ANOTHER SYMPTOM?

OF WHAT?

Reception

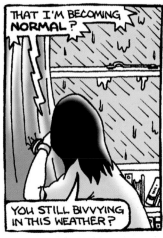

THAT I'M BECOMING **NORMAL**?

YOU STILL BIVVYING IN THIS WEATHER?

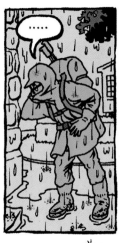

.....

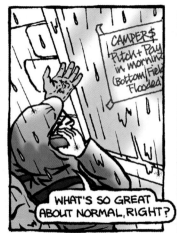

CAMPER$
Pitch + Pay
in morning
(Bottom Field
Flooded)

WHAT'S SO GREAT ABOUT NORMAL, RIGHT?

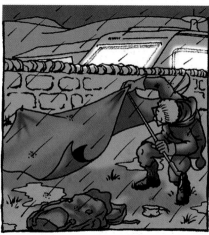

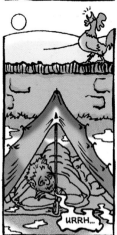

URRH...

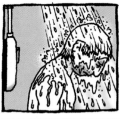

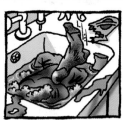

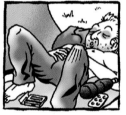

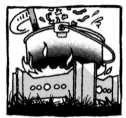

THREE DAYS LATER I WAS BACK ON TRACK.

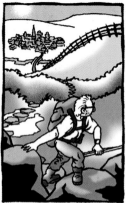

MAYBE I WAS LUCKY. MAYBE I FELL BETWEEN G.P.s, ESCAP-ED BEING BANGED UP IN HOSP-ITAL, WHACKED OUT ON MEDS.

ASIDE FROM LOOSE TEETH, SCREAMING TINNITUS AND A KNACKERED IMMUNITY SYSTEM WELCOMING BUGS, I HAD SURVIVED THE CHEMICAL ATTACK RELATIVELY UNSCATHED.

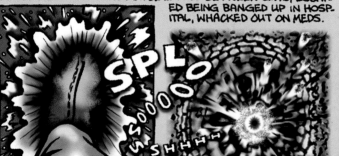

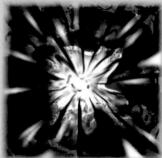

I STILL HAD THE MARBLES TO DOUBT MAD MEDICINE AND EXPLORE ALTERNA-TIVES TO THE WHITE MAN'S VOODOO.

YES, I STILL DUG DUNGEONS...

BUT NOW I OWNED THEM, GINGERLY EXPLORING THEIR FARTHEST CORNERS, RARELY REACHING DEAD ENDS.

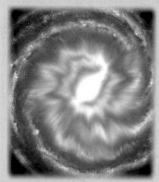

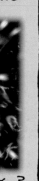

AND EMOTIONALLY...?

THERE WAS EVERY CHANCE I WOULD EMERGE MADDER THAN I WENT IN. THE CHALLENGE WAS HOW TO LIVE WITH INSANITY AND STAY SANE.

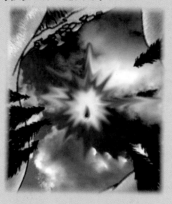

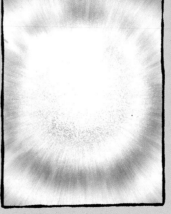

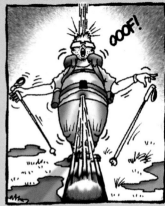

BUT I FOUND HOPE IN DARK PLACES. IT WAS IN THE LIGHT WHERE PROBLEMS PERSISTED.

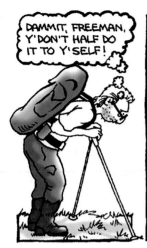

DAMMIT, FREEMAN, Y'DON'T HALF DO IT TO Y'SELF!

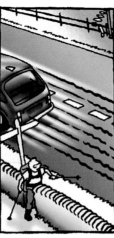

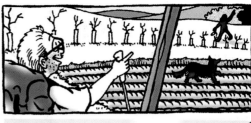

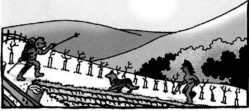

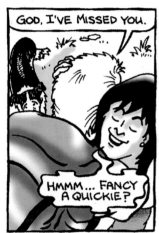

GOD, I'VE MISSED YOU.

HMMM... FANCY A QUICKIE?

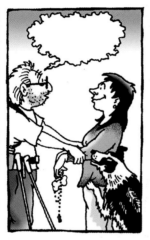

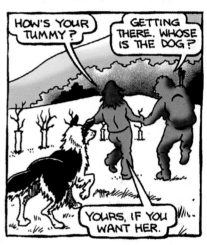

HOW'S YOUR TUMMY?

GETTING THERE. WHOSE IS THE DOG?

YOURS, IF YOU WANT HER.

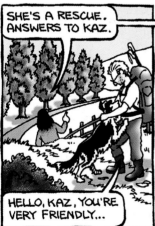

SHE'S A RESCUE. ANSWERS TO KAZ.

HELLO, KAZ, YOU'RE VERY FRIENDLY...

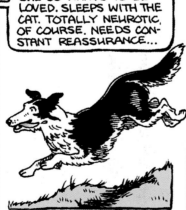

SHE SO WANTS TO BE LOVED. SLEEPS WITH THE CAT. TOTALLY NEUROTIC, OF COURSE. NEEDS CONSTANT REASSURANCE...

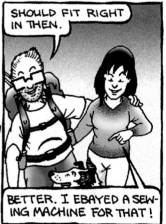

SHOULD FIT RIGHT IN THEN.

BETTER. I EBAYED A SEWING MACHINE FOR THAT!

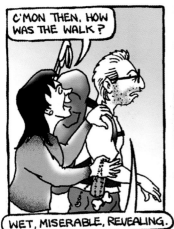

C'MON THEN, HOW WAS THE WALK?

WET, MISERABLE, REVEALING.

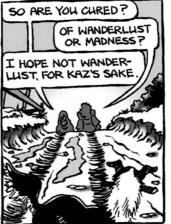

SO ARE YOU CURED?

OF WANDERLUST OR MADNESS?

I HOPE NOT WANDERLUST, FOR KAZ'S SAKE.

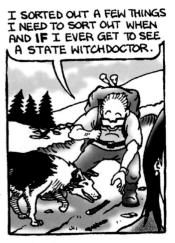

I SORTED OUT A FEW THINGS I NEED TO SORT OUT WHEN AND **IF** I EVER GET TO SEE A STATE WITCHDOCTOR.

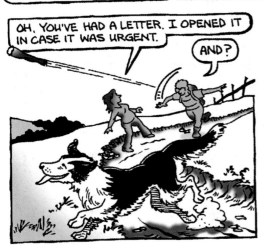

OH, YOU'VE HAD A LETTER. I OPENED IT IN CASE IT WAS URGENT.

AND?

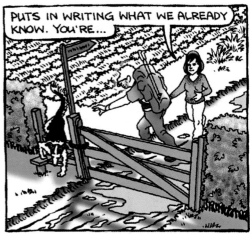

PUTS IN WRITING WHAT WE ALREADY KNOW. YOU'RE...

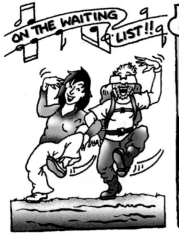

ON THE WAITING LIST!!

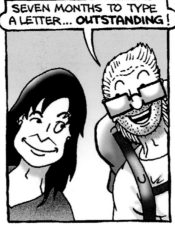

SEVEN MONTHS TO TYPE A LETTER... **OUTSTANDING**!

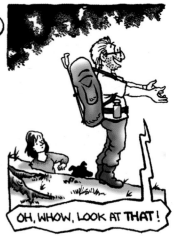

OH, WHOW, LOOK AT **THAT**!

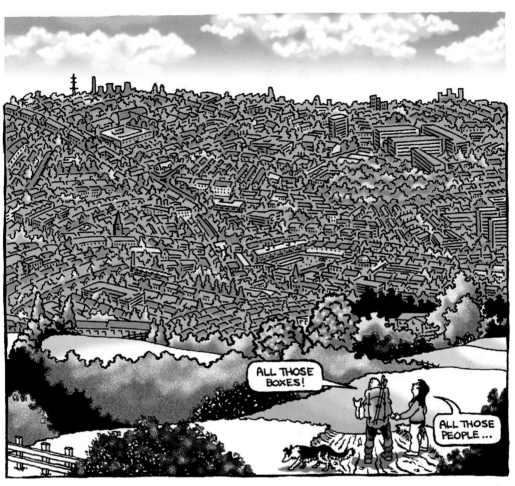

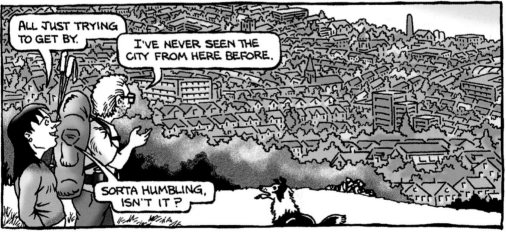

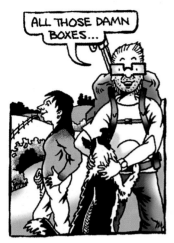

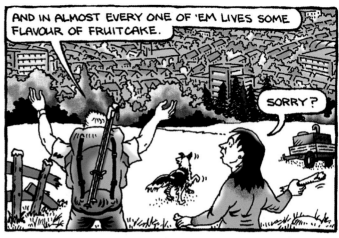

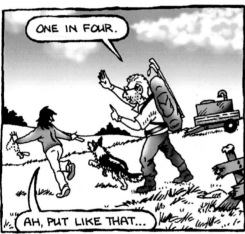

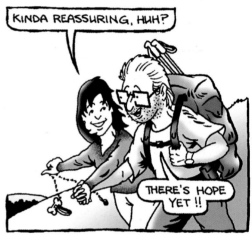

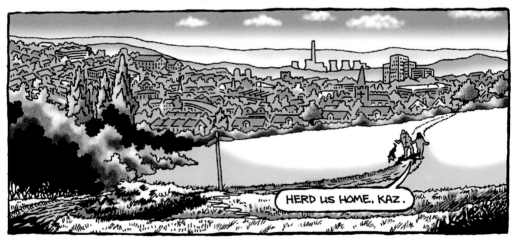

If you've been affected by any of the issues in this book, getta grip. It's only a comic!

Failing that, and before surrendering body and soul to GlaxoSmithKline, the following might be useful places to begin your journey:-

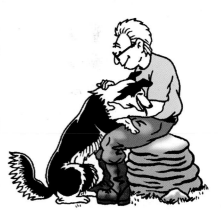

MIND -
www.mind.org.uk/help/information_and_advice

Open Up -
www.open-up.org.uk

Coming Off Psychiatric Medication -
www.comingoff.com

With enormous thanks to Ross, Myra, Helen and Making Waves in Nottingham, who helped me see white wasn't always black, and to Hunt, Knockabout and those I kick around with, who saw things I couldn't.

'Depresso' is by way of a deep apology to Sandy and Zoe, who got it in the neck every time.

Finally, let's hear it for the nerds who are still trying to catalogue the flicks I've referenced.

They are 2001: A Space Odyssey, Airplane, Brief Encounter, Wings of Desire, Yojimbo, Finding Nemo, Reservoir Dogs, Once Upon a Time in the West, Lawrence of Arabia, The Great Escape, The Third Man, North by Northwest, The Seventh Seal, The Birds, The Wizard of Oz, Singing in the Rain and Magical Mystery Tour.